6/23   7 2

THE LAST APPOINTMENT
Psychotherapy in General Practice

THE
LAST
APPOINTMENT

Psychotherapy
in General Practice

John Salinsky

The Book Guild Ltd.
Sussex, England

The Book Guild Ltd.
25 High Street,
Lewes, Sussex

First published 1993
© John Salinsky 1993
Typesetting by Southern Reproductions (Sussex)
East Grinstead, Sussex.
Printed in Great Britain by
Antony Rowe Ltd.
Chippenham, Wiltshire.

A catalogue record for this book is
available from the British Library

ISBN 0 86332 854 7

CONTENTS

To my brothers: Kenneth, who made the work possible, and Michael who led the way.

1

BEGINNINGS

For seventeen years I have been a General Practitioner. In a working day I see about forty patients, mostly in brief consultations lasting five to ten minutes. But on one or two days a week I also see a single patient for a long session of thirty or forty-five minutes at the end of the evening surgery. These patients are people with serious emotional problems whom I try to help by offering them a form of long term psychotherapy. I have been doing this for nearly all of my seventeen years as a GP and will probably continue to do so. Why have I found it necessary to add these extra, unpaid sessions to what is already a full day's work? I suppose because the patients appealed to me for help and I seemed to be the only person around who was willing and able to give them the kind of help that they needed.

I had been interested in psychoanalysis and psychotherapy since my discovery of Freud as an adolescent. When I was a medical student I intended to specialise in psychiatry and train as an analyst. But somehow I became disenchanted with Freud whose ideas, when I grew older, no longer seemed a totally satisfying explanation of all human behaviour. I became more interested in organic medicine and decided to become a hospital physician instead. However, the training for that speciality soon required me to do research and that meant spending too much time for my liking in the laboratory, studying basic disease processes. I came to the conclusion that I was more interested in talking to people than analysing their body fluids, and so I changed my mind again and opted for general practice. Here I discovered that many of the problems my patients brought me were emotional rather than physical. Some people felt tired all the time or lifeless, or miserable for no obvious reason. Others were full of fear about threats from the outside world or from within their own bodies. Some sufferers were quiet, likeable people who seemed to have been washed up on a desolate shore: unable to connect with anyone or to find any sense or purpose in their own lives.

With some of these troubled people I seemed to find a special sympathy or affinity. I liked them, I felt compassion for them, I wanted to help them. My interest in psychoanalysis was rekindled and I tried to find the explanations for their current problems in their childhood experiences. Sure enough, I would often unearth unhappy memories of cruelty and neglect; but simply recalling and retelling these experiences was not enough to provide the hoped-for cure. Much more was needed, and I felt that I had neither the time nor the skill to provide it. At first I tried to enlist the help of the psychiatric services; but I soon discovered that an appointment for the psychiatric clinic led nowhere. The consultant or registrar would provide forty-five minutes for the first interview, listen attentively, ask a lot of questions and then write a long report. But after he had reached a diagnostic formulation, his interest would recede rapidly and all he had to offer was a course of some anti-depressant or other. I knew that this might prove useless and had probably been tried already. I wanted my patients to have psychotherapy, but this was a very scarce commodity – except in the private sector which few of my patients could afford. In those days there were very few practice counsellors or clinical psychologists offering therapy. NHS psychotherapy, where it existed at all, took place mainly in groups which offered insufficient personal attention for my socially insecure deprived patients. A few clinics offered individual therapy, but this was mainly provided by doctors or therapists still in training and a rigorous selection interview ruled out any patient who might prove too difficult for a beginner to handle. Nearly all my patients failed this test; I was informed, apparently without conscious irony, that they were too ill to be suitable for treatment. So the patients came back to me, feeling rejected, hurt and disappointed. I shared in their disappointment and felt that as I was the only person in a position to help, untrained as I was, I had better get on with it.

I started inviting a few of these troubled people to book the last appointment of the evening surgery (6.30 pm) which would leave me free to spend up to an hour with them – at the cost of getting home late and rather tired. Had there been dozens of these patients I would soon have been overwhelmed. In fact I was fairly careful with my invitations and never took on more than three patients a week. Those I selected were always people for whom I felt a sort of special affinity: a mixture of liking, a desire to help and a feeling that here was somebody I could bear to sit with once a week for months or even years. They were not the easy cases by any means; anybody with a relatively simple problem I would refer to the real psychotherapists where, after a six month wait, they might get taken on. I was left with the people whom the professionals would not touch. Since I was the only chance they had, I did not feel that I was depriving them of the opportunity to be treated by someone more highly skilled.

Even so, in the early days, I worried about getting out of my depth. I had no training in psychotherapy; my only equipment was an interest in people and a basic knowledge of psychoanalytic theories gained from reading and from talking to friends in the trade. Suppose I actually made people worse? Perhaps I would cause them to have a breakdown. I was not too sure what that meant, but it did not sound good. Perhaps they would realise things about themselves that they could not cope with: they might go completely mad or commit suicide . . . It seemed a good idea to get some advice and the obvious person to approach was my elder brother, himself a GP but also a practising psychoanalyst.

My brother's help proved to be invaluable and he has continued to support and encourage me. Perhaps encouragement, or to use a jargon word, validation, was the first thing I needed. He actually thought that what I was trying to do was possible, worthwhile, and not dangerous. That was a great relief. Secondly, he taught me some basic principles of psychotherapeutic practice which had to do with the structure and the setting of the sessions rather than the content. He advised me to try to see each patient at the same time on the same day of the week and for exactly the same length of time. If the length of the session was set at forty-five minutes, (a useful sort of span: long enough to relax but not long enough to be exhausting) then it should always be forty-five minutes: no more and no less. This has the effect of making the patient feel that she has a space reserved for her which is constant and whose length does not depend on how interesting she has managed to be to her therapist that particular day. At the same time she is aware that at the end of forty-five minutes the therapist must be released to go home to her private life with her family. This may be difficult for the patient, but at least it sets a limit and prevents both patient and therapist from feeling that the therapist is in danger of being overworked and overwhelmed.

My brother also advised me to make an open-ended commitment to anybody I took on for these special sessions. This meant that the therapy was offered not for three months or a year but for as long as it was wanted. This is in complete contrast to the idea that setting a time limit serves to concentrate the patient's mind and encourages her motivation to 'get well' before the time runs out. This time limited approach may work for some people and it certainly enables a therapist to treat more patients. But I had already discovered that with the kind of people I was trying to help, the suggestion that we would stop after a given number of sessions only made them dread the ending and the rejection which that implied. Some psychotherapists would say that to go on indefinitely is to encourage 'dependent behaviour' and I can see their point. On the other hand, my patients seemed to have a desperate need for someone they could depend on for quite a long time. Only then could they begin to feel sufficiently secure in themselves to function without this kind of support.

A therapist engaged in this kind of emotionally demanding work also needs some support himself, and my brother provided this by offering me a monthly session to discuss my patients' progress with him. This enabled me to feel that I was not bearing all their pain and uncertainty alone and was less in danger of getting out of my depth or too involved without realising it. I was still without any experience of psychotherapy on the receiving end: that is of being a patient myself. Curiously enough, you need to know how to receive help if you are to provide it effectively for someone else, and most schools of psychotherapy regard personal therapy as an essential element of training. And so, after a few years, I decided to arrange for some psychoanalysis for myself. This was a considerable investment of time, money and faith, and deserves a chapter to itself. For the time being I shall say only that the experience did a great deal to make me more aware of my own feelings, and more open to the feelings of others. But this was still in the future. Meanwhile I wanted to make a start as a therapist.

With my brother's encouragement and support, I began to take on a number of patients for weekly sessions, usually of forty-five minutes, with an open-ended commitment. Some of these 'treatments', if that is the right word, ended after only a few months because the patients either moved away or found that it was not helping. Others went on for a number of years. With some patients the interval between sessions was extended to two or even four weeks by mutual agreement. I never saw anybody more than once a week and never took on more than three patients at a time. Even three is a little heavy and I am more comfortable with two weekly patients and perhaps one monthly. I could never take on a new patient unless I was sure that there was a vacancy. So the total number of my psychotherapy patients over seventeen years has been only about twenty. Not a great contribution to treating the psychopathology of even my small corner of the world, you may think, but at least I have been able to help a few people who would probably not have found that kind of help anywhere else.

What did my patients and I talk about in all those sessions? What sort of technique did I use? The answers may become clearer when I come to describe the individual patients and to tell their stories. First of all, I just listened to what they had to say – in itself very therapeutic. Then, in the early days, I made a lot of interpretations along psychoanalytic lines, as suggested by my reading and the advice of my brother. Nowadays I am not so sure that the kind of intellectual insight that you get from having your thoughts interpreted in the light of a particular theory of mental functioning is very helpful. I am more inclined to believe that the power of psychotherapy lies in the constancy of the relationship with the therapist as a person. Help comes, I think, from the feeling that someone reliable and concerned about you, is there to listen to you, feel with you, and even worry about you. That there is someone who cares about you for yourself and because you are her patient; not because you are clever, or amusing, or pretty or virtuous. If you achieve something good, your therapist will be pleased for you and with you – but you will still be her 'child' even if you do not win any prizes. I find myself using the model of parent and child to describe the relationship quite a lot in the interpretations I do make, because it is a good one, at least for me.

I see psychotherapy as a chance to replay childhood with a surrogate parent who will look after you and do her best for you, although she is human and will, from time to time, make mistakes, say the wrong thing or get upset. If the relationship between therapist and patient works, if the 'chemistry' is right, then the therapy will work too. Most of the process, in my view, is independent of the therapist's particular theoretical ideas. But the therapist may well need some sort of theoretical framework for her own support, just as a country priest needs some theology to sustain him in the care of his flock. I will return in a later chapter to questions of

13

doctrine, theory, relationships, chemistry and transference; I will also try to deal with the doubts that some
professional psychotherapists will have about the
advisability of my endeavours. But first, I think, I should
introduce some of the people I have worked with and
tried to help.

CASE HISTORIES

(The names of the patients in the following chapters have been altered in order to protect their anonymity)

2

DUNCAN

He was a tall, thin man in his late twenties when I first met him. He had a pale face with a high forehead and only a few wisps of dark hair left on the top of his head. His clothes were old and threadbare; his teeth were terrible – blackened, rotten and pointed. He was working as a railway booking clerk, was married and had two little girls. I think I had seen his wife and children already for various minor illnesses before he came to the surgery himself. I cannot remember what he wanted the first time he came, but fairly soon he must have started talking about how he was feeling depressed. I remember him telling me that he spent most of the night wandering about on a common, hoping that he would die of cold or exposure, because his life seemed so meaningless. He really wanted to be a writer and he had planned to go to university. At the time he was living in Australia, and that was what his parents wanted him to do. He passed matriculation and was accepted at an Australian university but instead of taking up his place, he suddenly decided to leave home, move to a small town a hundred miles away and get a job in a bank.

'Whenever I am about to succeed,' he said, 'I do something to make sure that I will fail.' In the small town

17

he met an Asian girl whom he wanted to marry. His parents were horrified, and came up with a plan to send him to university in Italy. Duncan thought this was simply to get him away from his girl. He refused, and his younger brother went to Italy in his place. Duncan came to England with Molly and they were married. 'By doing this,' he said, 'I made sure that I could not succeed in my real aim in life.'

He never used the word 'love' in talking about Molly – she seemed to be merely the instrument of his self destruction plan. 'She is not very intelligent,' he said, and added with typical arrogance, 'her IQ is about half mine.' When I met them, Duncan and Molly had been in England for about six years. During this time he had been working at several fairly undemanding jobs, ending up as a railway booking clerk. But he still had ambitions to go to a university and had managed to get one grade B pass in A-level English. The following year he studied history which he was good at; then after a few months he changed to maths, which he could not do and, predictably, he failed. Since then he had been studying French and German at home in his spare time; but lately he had lost his enthusiasm for studying. He was finding it difficult to concentrate on anything. Nothing seemed to be worthwhile. He felt unable to do anything unless he could think of a good reason. Some mornings he would lie in bed for hours because he could think of no good reason for getting up. He tended to forget things and was constantly making lists of things to be remembered. At work in the booking office he had a list of things to do which included 'sell tickets'. He was even afraid that he might completely forget the existence of Molly and the children unless he included their names on his list.

All this sounded very bizarre, but it was told in a quiet, slightly humorous way which I found appealing. I liked

18

him in spite of some of the weird things he was saying. He was obviously an intellectual and I felt that he needed to be rescued from his ticket office and his obsessional preoccupations so the he could go to university and become a writer. I was probably unaware of how seriously disturbed he was.

I asked him to come back and talk more, which he gladly agreed to do. On the next occasion I asked him about his childhood because I thought that there must be a clue there to his extraordinary self-defeating behaviour, and I was right. He had actually been born in England, the eldest child of middle-class parents (his father was a personnel officer). Then, when he was two years old, he was sent to live in Australia with his grandmother. The reason for this sudden uprooting of a two-year-old remains unclear, but he did not see his parents again for two years, although his grandmother kept assuring him that they were coming. When they did arrive, they brought with them a baby brother. Duncan did not speak of any jealousy of the new baby; he only remembered his parents being a disappointment and he continued to wait for the 'real' parents who he felt were still to come. Some sort of normal life with his parents was nevertheless established and two more children were born.

I was quite shocked at the insensitivity with which the two-year-old Duncan had been treated, and I felt sure that his problems all had their roots in this experience of loss and rejection at a time when he particularly needed affection and security from his parents. It explained his cool, detached, remote attitude to the world and to his own feelings. But where did we go from here? He appreciated the time I spent with him and my interest in his predicament. He had told me his life story and he could see how his treatment as an infant must have influenced his development. But seeing it did not make him feel any better. He still saw himself as a doomed, hopeless case.

I asssured him that this was not so (although I had no grounds other than my own hopefulness for doing so), and I arranged an appointment at a local and highly regarded centre for psychotherapy. They responded quickly and he had a number of interviews there with a medically qualified psychoanalyst and a clinical psychologist. Both agreed that he was suffering from 'a severe obsessional illness', and they wrote me a long account of all his obsessional symptoms. They mentioned his childhood separation from his parents and agreed that this was significant – but they did not see it as something on which work could be done, or as a wound which might be healed. They felt that Duncan's defences were elaborate but fragile: if they were penetrated he might be driven to suicide. In short there was 'no way in which he could be helped by analytic psychotherapy . . . it would stir up more conflicts than would be solved, almost certainly making him worse.' Instead, they suggested, he should be under the care of a general psychiatric clinic.

Duncan was disappointed by this rejection, but he agreed to referral to the general psychiatric department of the local hospital. Here he was offered some anti-depressant tablets (which he rejected) and a place in a therapy group (which he accepted). I had a long session with him in which we discussed his prospects and his general state of mind. He said that he wanted to achieve something really spectacular: like becoming a virtuoso pianist, or writing a masterpiece. 'I want to do something so big and so beautiful that it will completely absorb and enclose me.' But he also thought increasingly of suicide – as a spectacular achievement like that of Jan Palach, the

20

student who set fire to himself and became a martyr of the Czech uprising in 1968 (six years earlier). He noted that I remembered Jan Palach without difficulty; but many people who had known Duncan for six years had already forgotten about him. So he desperately wanted to be remembered (perhaps by that mother who was thousands of miles away when he was only two.)

I asked him why he was constantly telling me about his suicidal feelings. Was it to test whether I really cared? He said that talking about it prevented him from doing it. However, he had a friend who was always talking about suicide until his friends just got fed up with hearing about it and told him to go ahead and do it: so he killed himself. I told him that he was of value alive and that the world was diminished by any suicide. I wanted to give him some message to take away from that session that would neutralise his despair. He accepted the message graciously, and said that he was looking forward 'intellectually' to the first group therapy session. He would keep me in touch with his progress.

After that I saw him about every two months – and was given news of the group therapy. At first, it seems, he talked a good deal there, and helped to get things moving. Later, when other people had more to say about themselves, he began to feel isolated and to feel that he had little to offer. Then he began missing sessions. After missing three in a row he felt reluctant to go back because he did not believe that the others still cared about him. In the end he did return, but only for a few weeks before dropping out permanently. After that he wrote me a letter which I still have in my files. It is dated 24th of May 1976 (about two years after we first met). In it he says, 'I have made a complete mess of everything including my plans for university. My wish now is that no more time should be wasted on me. It is pointless. I am not ungrateful for all that has been done, but all I want to do now is to stop thinking, and above all, I do not want to talk to anyone. I have managed to let down a lot of people and there is no way I can ever make up for that. I know that that was my last chance to break out.'

I was very moved by this letter and felt that I wanted to offer to help him personally as well as I could. I wrote to him offering to see him for a long session once a week at a time to be arranged to suit us both. He accepted my offer, and the four years of weekly 'therapy' began.

THE WEEKLY SESSIONS

We had some difficulty in finding a suitable time for the sessions. I wanted to give Duncan a full hour (although the analysts say that fifty minutes is enough – perhaps to give them ten minutes to collect their thoughts between cases.) I was already seeing other people at the end of the surgery on two nights a week and that seemed enough. His shift work in the booking office also made it difficult to find a regular afternoon slot. Instead we settled for six p.m. on a Saturday, which sounds very awkward, but actually suited me quite well. If I was going out on the Saturday evening, if left me enough time, and it was nicely separated from the rest of the working week. I did not feel that my weekend was being unduly encroached on. All the same, I must have felt on the first occasion that we needed a little sustenance because I took along two cans of lager which we solemnly sipped as we talked. The following week Duncan brought the drinks and we continued to alternate for some weeks. My brother (and supervisor) disapproved of these refreshments because, he said, Duncan would have unconscious fantasies of me as a feeding mother which would become contaminated by reality if I was actually feeding him with lager during the sessions. He did not press this objection too strongly and after a while the custom was allowed to lapse anyway.

I have mentioned my brother's advice about keeping the sessions going in a regular pattern and I think it was particularly important for Duncan to know that I was going to see him every week, except for holidays, and that the appointed hour was his for as long as he needed it. There were occasional variations of the time and the day, (Sunday instead of Saturday) to fit in with his shift work or my social life. He missed only a few sessions, generally due to misunderstanding about a change of time (no doubt unconsciously motivated!) One week I asked him to come at eight p.m. I arrived at the surgery five minutes early, released the catch on the back door, (our usual arrangement) and waited in my consulting room for him to let himself in. I waited for about half an hour by which time it was clear that he was not coming. The next day he telephoned to say that he had come at seven o'clock and again at nine o'clock.

On another occasion I completely forgot about a six o'clock session. At eight o'clock I suddenly remembered, and felt that I had let him down terribly. I telephoned at once and offered to go round to his house to save him from having to walk to the surgery in the rain. My lapse did not result in any deterioration in our relationship – it seemed to improve as a result. He seemed to find the whole experience of being let down and then picked up again quite elating; and the fact that I was prepared to come round to his house confirmed that I was genuinely concerned about his welfare.

I have emphasised the importance of regularity in the sessions; of keeping the same day, same hour and same duration of sessions because of the feeling of security which this provides for the patient. And yet, against a steady background of regular sessions, the interruptions, the occasions when things go wrong and appointments are missed, are even more important. I think that Duncan's picture of the world of relationships was one in which promises were rarely kept and if people let him down, they were not particularly sorry about it, and did not attempt to make good the damage. In his case, exile to Australia at the age of two, probably initiated this bleak view of human nature.

One evening, when the weekly therapy had been going on for about three years, Duncan rang up in a state of some distress about his elder daughter, aged six, who had some kind of feverish illness. He only wanted advice over the telephone but I offered to visit and he gratefully accepted. She was not seriously ill, and I was able to reassure the whole family that she only had flu and would soon be better. It was an ordinary home visit of which, like every GP, I do several hundred in a year. But for Duncan it seemed to have a special meaning. In the session which followed, he expressed his thanks and seemed much more willing to trust me than he had been before. It was as though by demonstrating my willingness to care for his child I had shown him that I could be relied on to care for, and care about, the child part of him.

What did we talk about during the sessions? We talked a good deal about how he saw himself (usually with gloom and dismay). He felt that the combination of parental genes and unfortunate experiences in early childhood had damaged him permanently, and that the struggle to improve was probably futile. We also discussed his attitude to the therapy and his relationship with me. Often he saw me as a competitor, an antagonist or even a superior chess player. Perhaps this was due to my tendency to reply to his offerings with 'clever' interpretations (some of which he would learn to predict in advance). However he also acknowledged that I was spending a lot of time with him for which I was not being paid. For a time he speculated on what might be in it for me. Was I enjoying the chess game? Was I acting out of high-minded charity? Or was I really trying to help him because I cared about what happened to him? My interpretations, usually in terms of a child and parent model, would lead him to talk about his parents and his own children. I would then make comparisons between his care of his own children and my looking after the child part of him. When he was silent after a holiday break, I might suggest that 'the infant part of him' was unwilling to feed from my breast, which his own projected anger had turned into a hostile breast. When he talked about feeling as if he was being questioned by two interrogators, one sympathetic, the other hostile, I said that this was a child's view of the parents apparently antagonistic, but secretly collaborating (in sexual intercourse).

Some of these ideas (deriving from the work of Melanie Klein) he found interesting; sometimes they seemed to fit with his own ideas – more often they only reinforced his feeling that I was cleverer than he was. On one occasion he floored my by saying cunningly, 'If I were to pronounce the words "Melanie Klein", what effect would that have on you?' (Subsequently my brother reassured me that it was all right and could only be helpful for the patient to read the source books as well as the therapist). All these interpretations came to my mind very freely, not only from my own reading of Mrs Klein but from two other psychoanalytical influences that were operating on me at the time. Firstly, I was discussing Duncan's progress with my brother once a month and being fed with his Kleinian interpretations about what was going on in the sessions. And secondly, I was having my own (Kleinian) analysis for most of the period during which I was seeing Duncan, so I found it easy and natural to reproduce the kind of language I was used to hearing from my analyst.

Looking back on my attempts to be a pretend analyst for Duncan I am inclined to think that my interpretations were pretty inept and inaccurate, but I do not think that they did him any harm. And I needed some sort of theoretical framework to cling to while I held on to Duncan and prevented him from being washed away. The Kleinian model happened to be the one I knew best and felt most at home with. But any changes that happened in Duncan's mind and in his life had more to do with the fact that I held on to him for four years, than to any insights he may have gained from my second-hand interpretations.

In any case, our discourse was not restricted to attempts at decoding what he had to say. On a more practical level, we also talked about his physical health and, in particular, his awful teeth and his phobia about going to the dentist. Lastly we talked about his plans for the future: whether he would be able to get two more good A-level grades, leave the ticket office, and go to a university. Here is a sample of one of our later sessions taken from the notes which I made at the time:

Silence. Then he said, 'I think you hit the right note last week. But you might not hit it again so easily. The same one might not be right this week in any case.' I asked what he meant. He said, 'If I could really communicate the way I feel, it would change you quite a lot, but it would not affect me.' I said that he seemed to be telling me that he was powerful and dangerous. 'Anger and hatred is all I have,' he said. 'Take that away and there would be nothing.' I said I was interested in what he was angry about.

There was a long silence in which he seemed to go to sleep several times and wake up with a jerk. I said that his silence made me feel shut out, helpless, powerless to do anything. Was this a feeling he wanted me to have instead of him? He said he did feel helpless and perhaps shut out. More silence. I felt irritated. I asked if he really wanted to come any more. He said he did. Somehow, the sessions kept him going during the week – prevented the pain from rising over the threshold and becoming unbearable. Although it might be better if the pain did rise and knocked him out altogether. Meanwhile, he went through life trying to minimise discomfort. I said that when he did come to see me he sat there not telling me how it felt – perhaps to avoid more discomfort and pain. 'It is the only event of the week,' he said, 'coming here. I need an event. Otherwise I am a complete non-person. That is what I am trying to become. Have not yet succeeded. Something in me makes me go on living.'

This all sounds very bleak and despairing. Reading it again, I wonder how I retained any hope. I think I had a sense that the rhythm of the sessions, the regular 'event of the week', was keeping him going, keeping a spark alive. My brother's encouragement was also important in enabling me to keep the sessions going without getting too agitated about how I was going to bring about any change in Duncan.

And yet he did change. Very gradually, with many false dawns and relapses back into darkness. He began to admit (grudgingly at first) that he had some feeling of trust for me as well as feelings of suspicion, competition, envy and so forth. As I have said, the trust was fostered as much by the events which happened outside the sessions and which told him I was trying to care for him and was

27

feeling some responsibility for him. I am thinking of my home visit to his little daughter and the occasion when I visited his house to make up for a missed session. Indications that I was a real person and not just someone playing a therapeutic chess game were always helpful – but only against a background of regular sessions extending indefinitely into the future.

The most impressive change over the four years of weekly meetings was the way in which he managed to work for his A-levels and overcome his reluctance to expose himself to the examiners' judgment. In June 1978, he was able to tell me that he had done the French A-level papers without missing any, and without walking out half way through (which he had done more than once in previous years.) 'It seemed less trouble to stay than to walk out this time,' was his characteristic way of putting it. He must have put some work into those papers because he was given a grade B, with which he was very pleased.

The following academic year he began studying German with the help of another patient of mine who came from Austria. There were still plenty of gloomy sessions in which his mood was almost suicidal. Others were a little more lively and there was generally a ration of his sardonic humour to help keep both of us going. He began to apply to universities. One of them asked for a report on his emotional problems which he had described as interrupting his academic career. The Admissions Tutor was concerned about his ability to cope with the rigours of an Honours degree course. I was able to reply that he had made considerable progress with his difficulties and that I thought he had the necessary motivation to carry him through. In the summer of the fourth year of our weekly sessions, he duly sat the German examinations and gained another B grade.

He was accepted with these grades by two universities and, after some difficulty, he chose one of them. We then spent a lot of time discussing practical problems: where were he and the family going to live? (They now had a third child, a little boy). How would they afford it? Would he have to give up smoking? What would happen to the cat? Should he brave the dentist and get his teeth fixed?

Happily he managed to find a little house in a village not far from the campus, where there was room for them all at a very low rent. A couple of painful dental abscesses precipitated a visit to the dentist whose verdict was that all his teeth would have to come out. He managed to go through this ordeal too and emerged looking much more presentable, with a set of false teeth – which he seemed to adapt to very quickly. As the summer drew to its end we began to talk about saying goodbye. He acknowledged that he might miss having me to talk to once a week but he was not able to say 'I shall miss you'. That would have meant lowering his defences too much, and I did not expect it. Instead, he and Molly held a little party to say thank you to all his helpers – including me and the people who had given him coaching in French and German. It was a pleasant evening and he talked eagerly about his plans for the future.

He sent me a Christmas card from college that year, indicating briefly that all was going well. The following summer I accepted his invitation to visit them for the weekend in the village, about a hundred miles away, where they now lived. They all welcomed me warmly and told me how good the local people had been in helping them to settle in. Molly seemed content that Duncan was at last doing what he wanted to do and the children were enjoying the freedom of living in the country. Duncan

29

showed me round the university and told me that he was enjoying academic life and having no problems in keeping up with the work. We had a couple of beers in the pub; we took the children to the seaside for the afternoon; we talked about literature and life in general, but neither of us referred to the therapy or its relationship to his new way of life. It seemed better to leave it unspoken.

A year later I received a heart-rending letter from Molly. She told me that Duncan was having an affair with a female lecturer at the University and had gone to spend a year studying in Germany with her. She was planning to take the children back to Australia to join her family. She said she hoped I and my family were well, and that we would meet again some day. 'Life is very hard for me at present, but we must hope for better times to come.' Poor Molly. It seemed that I had not really done her a favour by helping Duncan to 'fulfil his potential'.

Since then I have not heard from either of them and several more years have passed. Writing this makes me wonder what has happened to Duncan. I like to think that he has done well academically (as though he were really one of my children), but I also fear that he may have been overwhelmed by that inner despair of his and committed suicide. It would be good to hear from him again.

3

MARGARET

I first met Margaret ten years ago. For nine of those years we have been having regular psychotherapy sessions in an unbroken sequence – first weekly, then monthly for a short, uncomfortable time. Then back to weekly, then fortnightly, three weekly, monthly and, for the last year, once every five weeks. Several times I have tried to bring the sessions to an end because I thought we were getting nowhere and wasting my time. But Margaret knew better, and she refused to let me go while she still had need of me. She has need of me still, but the urgency and desperation are no longer there, and I imagine that the interval will go on gradually lengthening until she no longer needs me.

Not far from my surgery there is a rather weird, Gothic looking house which is used by the local authority social services as a hostel for patients who have been discharged from the psychiatric hospital but are still too emotionally fragile to find a place of their own. I had recently agreed to be the GP for this hostel (which has up to six residents) and to look after the general medical needs of anyone who came to live there. The residents were usually sad, isolated, and occasionally, mad, people who came to me mainly to renew their prescriptions for anti-depressants or anti-psychotic drugs and to be certificated for invalidity benefit.

Margaret was one of them. She was thirty-three years old, quite tall, thin, angular and slightly stooping with a nose which was red and bleak in cold weather. She had slightly wavy fair hair and generally dressed in an anorak or sweater and wide trousers of a kind which played down or even denied her femininity. Her gaze was generally directed at the floor; her demeanour was mournful and despondent. She brought with her a letter of introduction from her (male) social worker. He said that she was depressed, socially isolated, slightly paranoid and lacking in confidence because of her homosexuality. He had been giving her individual therapy sessions for over a year but had now discontinued them 'because I feel that she needs to cope with the depression herself.'

In the first three months, she came to the surgery about once a week, seeing sometimes me, sometimes one of my partners. She would complain of depression or feelings that people at work were looking at her with contempt. At other times she would have physical symptoms such as stomach pain, poor appetite, nausea or weakness. She also referred angrily to some therapy at the hospital which had 'gone wrong' in a way that made her feel hurt and rejected. Despite these problems she was working steadily as an accounts clerk and arranging to transfer from the hostel to her own rented flat. After she moved into this flat, we did not see Margaret for nine months. Then she returned in a state of high agitation with her old symptoms intensified. She could not talk to anyone at work, people were laughing at her everywhere, she was terrified of becoming schizophrenic, she cried all the time, she was drinking. . . I calmed her down with the help of some tablets and she came back to see me every few days for the next fortnight while we pieced together her story.

MARGARET'S STORY

She was the third child in a family of four. Her father was a long distance lorry driver who was away a good deal of the time; but she remembered being his favourite when she was about nine. After that he began to come into the bedroom, where she shared a bed with her elder sister, and attempt to fondle her sister sexually. Both girls were frightened and begged him to stop, but he persisted. He threatened them with punishment if they told their mother what was going on, and neither of them did. Margaret was afraid of upsetting her mother, but felt guilty for not telling her. Their father's abusing behaviour stopped after about a year, but Margaret hated him after that and he grew very cold towards her. She became a nervous child, afraid to go to school without her mother, afraid even to go out in the rain.

At some time in her mid-teens she had a breakdown, which she remembers only dimly, but it was the beginning of a series of bouts of depression, overdoses, visits to perplexed doctors and social workers, long periods in hospital and episodes of therapy of one sort or another. She seems to have spent many hours in therapeutic groups, a lonely and pathetic figure, desperate for care and attention. None of her therapeutic relationships seem to have gone on long enough; she would begin to feel a little more secure in a hospital therapy group and then, suddenly, she would be discharged.

Her pleas to have the treatment extended or renewed met with temporising or firm rejection. Many times she was told that she must learn to manage on her own, but always she came back for more help, frightened and hungry. Her most recent period in hospital had at first seemed more hopeful. For eighteen months she had lived in a special villa at the hospital where the patients lived together as a community, and had therapy both collectively and individually. Some of them, including Margaret, had jobs outside the hospital, but returned there in the evenings and at weekends. During this time Margaret began to feel a sexual attraction towards women, who had always seemed to offer greater warmth and affection since her alienation from her father (who refused to have anything to do with Margaret after she became 'mentally ill'.)

Her therapist at the hospital was a sympathetic woman social worker called Ursula who gave Margaret a lot of time and encouragement. Margaret grew increasingly attached to Ursula and eventually fell in love with her. Whether one regards this as real love or an erotic transference does not, I think, really matter. It was real enough to Margaret, and Ursula seems at first to have responded warmly – and incautiously. According to Margaret, Ursula reassured her that homosexuality was nothing for a woman to be ashamed of, and revealed that she herself was homosexual. Margaret interpreted this as meaning that Ursula was in love with her too, and this impression was probably reinforced by the hugs and kisses which she gave Margaret from time to time during their sessions. However, when it became clear that Margaret was seriously in love with her, Ursula seems to have panicked and run to her supervisor, who quickly intervened and told poor Margaret that her therapy with Ursula had been terminated. No explanations were given or, at least, none that made any sense to Margaret. She was due to be discharged to the hostel in any case and, instead of continuing sessions with Ursula, she was allocated to a male social worker who had the difficult job of containing the damage while defending the decision of his hospital colleagues.

Eighteen months after her separation from Ursula, Margaret still felt puzzled, hurt and betrayed. She had also lost most of the inner security she had gained from Ursula's work with her in the hospital. This was the state she was in when I first met her. After the first flurry of anxiety she seemed to settle down for a while (with the help of her new social worker), and I think her return to the surgery was precipitated by his leaving to take up another post.

I remember looking at Margaret as she sat drooping in front of me and thinking that she looked like a large, awkward child who felt that she was an object of ridicule to everyone. It seemed unlikely that any other therapist would be willing to take her on; and something about her helplessness must have touched me and made me decide to offer her a regular session. I knew by that time that six months or a year would not be enough. But I could not have predicted that we would still be together nine years later.

WEEKLY THERAPY – THE FIRST PHASE

The first phase lasted for three years. We agreed that she would come on Wednesday evenings for forty-five minutes at the end of surgery. At first she was quite apprehensive, wanting to please me but not sure if she could trust me. She had, after all, been let down by several of my predecessors, for one reason or another. She talked about feeling angry with herself for being 'immature and childish'; as if childhood for her meant

35

only scorn and humiliation. This was the stage when she told me about her father and also about Ursula whom she said she loved more than anyone else. She believed that Ursula had loved her too, until she checked herself and withdrew into her professional detachment.

Then she told me about her discovery that she was a lesbian. 'You do not need to worry about me getting hooked on you,' she said. But I was not really convinced about her sexual preference. Her attachments to women seemed to be more to do with her need for warmth and affection and belonging rather than anything sexual. She had a girl-friend called Lorna with whom she had some tentative physical contacts; but it did not really seem to be right for either of them. When I suggested that her declaration of her homosexuality was really a way of dismissing men and making them feel unwanted, she sensed a disapproval of female homosexuality of any kind in my attitude and told me that I was a strict moralist ('like my father') and not free and easy like her previous therapists. However, she did admit that she found the women in the gay bars she occasionally ventured into a little strange and 'mixed up.'

Eventually Lorna disengaged herself from Margaret, who cried a little when she told me about it. She wondered if I was glad because I 'disapproved' of her relationship with Lorna anyway. The following week she came so late that I had given up and gone home. We sorted this out on the telephone and when she came on time the following week she said she was angry with me, but also afraid that I would get fed up with her like Lorna and Ursula. I tried to explain that I was more patient than that and that I thought she needed someone who would stay with her whether she was nice to them or not. This seemed to go down well, but the following week she was again 'disillusioned' with me because I had not waited for her two weeks earlier when she was late. Margaret was a great one for keeping her reproaches smouldering away like hot coals for extended periods. Now she said that she did not like the idea of my having a wife and family to go home to, if my patients appeared not to be turning up.

We talked about her jealousy as a child when everyone: father, sister and younger brother seemed to be coming between her and her mother. This discussion seemed to make her feel a little better. Margaret always liked plenty of interpretations, perhaps because she had been well steeped in psychotherapy before she came to me, and found them comforting. Later on, when my style became gradually simplified and I made fewer interpretations she complained about the lack of them – unlike some of my other patients for whom interpretations were an unnecessary irritation.

One interpretation that she did find disturbing was the suggestion that she might have felt jealous of the physical affection involved in her parents' sexual life together. I was prompted to introduce this idea because she said she found it painful even to think of me having a private life that she knew nothing about. After that she tended to be silent and sulky at the beginning of our sessions, perhaps trying (successfully) to make me be the one who had to attract attention. But then she would find it difficult to say anything at all in reply to my overtures, and begin to fear that I was losing interest in her. Eventually, when this fear came to light, I reassured her that I thought she was making some progress and I had no plans to end the sessions (although this would not always be true as we shall shortly see).

Having convinced herself that she was about to get the sack, Margaret now said that she felt relieved that I was still going to be her therapist. She followed this up with a backhander, saying she wondered whether I really was any good as a therapist, and perhaps I was just using her to practice on? A little later, she decided that being able to trust me was the most important thing. She told me how her father used to comfort her when her mother was preoccupied with the baby; how she loved him, and how he had broken her heart when he started interfering with her and her sister.

In the next session she began to speculate about an embryonic relationship with the man next door whom she had invited in for coffee. She wondered if she could cope with a boyfriend – would she have to wear make-up and look feminine like her mother? It seemed to me very likely that this talk about a man friend referred at least partly to me, but I kept that to myself, not wishing to embarrass her. At the end of that session she was reluctant to go and complained that the sessions were not long enough. All the same, she said, my strictness about timekeeping had the advantage that she knew where she was: Ursula used to run over time and sometimes gave her extra sessions. 'It was chaotic.'

In the next few sessions I heard more details about life at home with her parents. In particular, I learned about the terrible day when her mother came home unexpectedly and found her father sexually fondling Margaret's sister. Her mother said if it happened again she would have to send both girls away. Margaret would not kiss her father goodnight after that; then she stopped kissing her mother as well because he felt unfairly treated.

She painted a dark picture of her parents' marriage: they seemed always to be having rows, and her father was always either 'mauling' her mother or hitting her. I believed that it could not have been as bad as all that, but now I am not so sure. I was very much under the spell of the Kleinian picture of family life in which the parents behave like sensible, loving adults amd the children's minds are full of jealous, murderous, fantasies, wanting the parents' time together to be violent and unhappy. How can one tell what it was really like? Certainly her father had been very embittered and had refused to speak to Margaret or even have her in the house when he was there for many years after her breakdown. She would have to spend Christmas at her sister's, and her mother would slip out to join them for part of the day, leaving the old man at home.

As Christmas approached we prepared for a holiday break, and she asked how long I thought the treatment would go on for altogether. I said I thought about three years, which seemed a reasonably generous amount of my time to offer her. Margaret said that she might not be better in three years: then I would be disappointed and feel that I had wasted my time. I said that I might be disappointed but I would not feel the time had been wasted. Again, she seemed to draw some comfort from that.

The following year was quite a stormy one for our relationship. Margaret came back from the Christmas break feeling angry with me for making her feel dependent on me and miss me. Then she started to feel guilty about saying ungrateful things to me; she was even afraid of me, and afraid that I would be dissatisfied with her progress and terminate the sessions. After that she became so obviously depressed that I gave her some anti-depressant tablets to take. Then she veered from depression back to anger. I was mocking her by referring to her not just as a child but as a baby!

I explained as carefully as I could that I thought these chaotic feelings about me had their origin in her infancy and her baby feelings about her parents. I think now that she probably feared being as helpless as a baby, unable to do without me, crying for me when I was not there. She said: 'I used to telephone Ursula up from the ward all the time; I do not want to go through all that with you.' She wished I would not try to go so fast, put pressure on her, give her such a hard time. 'You used to be so supportive and reassuring. My other therapists were always sympathetic and understanding.'

Now and then she went to see a woman social worker at a day centre, whom she had known for some time. This social worker was more comforting than me. 'She makes me feel better when you make me feel worse.' Somehow I coped with the anger and the reproaches and the grudges nursed for weeks at a time. Occasionally she would apologise 'to the nice part of you that is trying to help.' I thought that sounded as though I was a mixture of a nice mother and a horrible father. Margaret agreed. But she added that Mother seemed to need Father – she was frightened when he was away for the night and had to have one of the girls sleep with her.

After Easter, we entered a more cheerful period in which we could discuss these ideas without them seeming so painful: although she still felt 'choked' if I said that Father had a special place in Mother's affections. The summer holidays were a more difficult time. She went away with a group of people but still felt isolated, and lonely; a figure of fun as far as the others were concerned. The friend she went with had a boyfriend and proximity to this loving couple painfully increased her feelings of jealousy and exclusion. The holiday was a disaster, but once it was over her self confidence gradually began to improve. She joined a tennis club and started going to dances. She felt less depressed but it was always an effort to keep a social conversation going – she preferred just to listen to people who talked a lot about themselves.

THE CRISIS AND THE SECOND PHASE

Time went by and the weekly sessions continued.
Margaret continued to make progress. She was working
steadily without having to be absent for sickness; she had
a reasonable social life for a single person, and she had
recently joined a local church which promised further
social and even spiritual opportunities. But she still felt
'low' or 'flat' for most of the time, despite her anti-
depressants. She had no close friends and nobody to love
her except her mother and nobody to care for her except
June, the social worker and, of course, me.

As for me, the three years I promised were coming to
an end, we seemed to have gone about as far as we could
go, Margaret seemed unlikely to change any further and I
thought it was time to stop. I realised that a complete
break would be more than she could cope with and we
agreed on a reduction of the sessions to once a
month.

In the next few weeks we talked about parting as if we
would never see each other again. She tried very hard to
develop a social life in the church to fill the gap but was
upset when the minister's wife silently handed her a book
about how to deal with 'Tension.' Our last weekly session
was painful. She told me I was enjoying the fact that the
sessions were ending. It is true that I was looking forward
to having a longer respite between sessions from a
patient who had become a fairly heavy burden to bear,
but I still cared for her.

We had four monthly sessions, all of which were fairly
painful, the air heavy with Margaret's resentment at
being downgraded. Had it not been for the support she

received from June, the social worker, I do not think she would have survived for so long. In the fourth session, I told her that she could telephone me at home if she really needed to, but she said she would never have the courage. On the following day, she found the courage, and used the opportunity to call me (among other things) 'a rotten bastard.' We had a session after that in which Margaret cried and seemed to get a little relief; but it did not last. She appeared at the surgery a few days later looking ill and ragged. Her speech was slurred and she talked in a jumbled way about thinking she was her father, and hearing her family talking to her in her head or through the walls of her flat. I was very alarmed and arranged an emergency appointment with a psychiatrist who thought that her extreme distress had spilled over into a psychotic kind of illness. She was started on a fairly heavy regime of anti-psychotic drugs and after a few days the bizarre symptoms subsided. She managed to avoid admission to hospital. I felt very responsible for the whole episode since my severe rationing of myself had clearly precipitated the crisis. The obvious remedy was to reinstate the weekly sessions: but with whom? And for how long? The psychiatrist was in no doubt about either question: 'You've got her for life!' she told me, cheerily.

I saw Margaret again and offered her a weekly session for half an hour instead of forty-five minutes. It seemed a bit mean, but I felt I needed to be able to get home a bit earlier if I was going to survive. She accepted the offer very readily and, with this new phase of treatment, introduced a new problem. She had become very troubled by a sort of compulsion to look at people's groins and imagine what their genital organs looked like. In particular, she was obsessed by the thought of men's genitals, hiding behind their trouser fronts. She would stare at a man's trousers for a long time and then begin to feel that the man had noticed the direction of her gaze, making her feel terribly embarrassed and ashamed.

She began asking me questions about genitalia and male sexuality, almost like a child seeking this kind of information for the first time. What were boys' nipples like, she asked me, and did they ever secrete milk? She remembered being in hospital for a tonsillectomy when she was seven and wondering whether some marks on her groins meant that she once had testicles. She also thought about couples a good deal; what their bodies looked like and what they did together. She sometimes thought men were lucky because they could feed from their wives' breasts. This thought also embarrassed her if she thought that the couple in question might be reading her mind.

I contributed a few interpretations about children and parents' sexuality, but I think they were really superfluous. The important thing was she was able to trust me with these questions and revelations without feeling embarrassed and foolish. She told me about her one sexual relationship with a man which had occurred when she was twenty-five. He was always pawing her and trying to get her into bed but she did not really enjoy the sex and soon broke it off because his demands were so tiresome. She missed him for a few months but then it wore off. 'I cannot cope with men – they want it all the time – cannot restrain themselves – it is such a bore. If you were married your bed would never be your own.'

Then the focus shifted to religion. She wanted to know if I believed in God and what my religion was. She imagined my family being religious and going to church, or perhaps a synagogue if I was Jewish. I said I did not follow any religion, but I thought that ideas about God

43

were important. It emerged that Margaret believed that when you died you went straight to hell if you did not believe in Jesus. This was what the minister of her church said and she had no reason to doubt it. She agreed that this was a frightening view of God and hard to reconcile with the idea of a loving, merciful, forgiving God. 'But my father was like that: he used to say "Do as I say, or go to hell." ' He would not put up with Margaret being ill or feeling depressed; never forgave her for it, apparently. In the end she decided to leave the church and to abandon the fundamentalist beliefs that went with it. For a while she was afraid that the minister would seek her out and ask her why she had stopped coming on Sundays, but he never did.

She described a lot of dreams during this period; they were all recorded carefully in a notebook and it was evidently important not to miss any out. Their themes included weddings, family gatherings, horoscopes, a woman 'on the shelf', being stranded in Germany without a passport, someone having a baby, and a pickpocket in a crowd. I did not really know what they meant and was, by then, a less enthusiastic provider of interpretations. But I think that she needed to show me that she had some interesting things to say, and the dreams did enable her to tell me, by means of associations, about her jealousy of my family life and my holidays.

Fifteen months after the psychotic breakdown, we agreed to reduce the sessions to once every two weeks and this transition was managed without disaster. I used the idea of a baby growing up and becoming first a toddler, then a schoolchild; gradually feeling confident enough to spend longer and longer periods away from her mother. After another year, we extended the interval to three weeks. After much trepidation, Margaret joined a social club for single people which organised country walks, theatre outings and trips to stately homes. This proved to be a great success, and provided her with a much needed way of meeting people and extending her interests. Our sessions became quiet, supportive and uneventful. She seemed to be finding life bearable, but she still felt disappointed that she had never really changed from the lonely, vulnerable, apprehensive 'flat' person she had been since her adolescence. I had to agree that further change seemed very unlikely. And then the miracle happened.

THE MIRACLE

Four years had passed since the psychotic crisis. The sessions were down to once a month and holding. Then Margaret made an appointment halfway through the month and told me she wanted me to give her some special sessions of forty-five minutes (instead of the usual thirty) to help her with her 'sexual identity.' She thought that I had helped her with her feelings about her mother but I had now become like her father. She was afraid of her anger towards me and wanted to understand it better.

(I remembered that in the previous two sessions she had linked hatred for her father with anxiety about her own sexual feelings. She had expressed her anger with men for thinking about sex all the time and 'forcing themselves into women.') So we agreed to have six forty-five minute sessions on Margaret's sexual identity (although I still was not sure what she meant by 'identity'.)

The first session was all about sex and her father and did not seem to me to break any new ground. But at the second session (a month later) she announced that she had been to a dance, started a conversation with a man 'in a cuddly jumper' and had later had him round to her flat for 'a nice sex-free evening.' He was a bachelor in his forties, rather shy like her, but comfortable to be with.

I held my breath, waiting for something to go wrong. But nothing went wrong. Their relationship flowered and most of the subsequent 'sexual identity' sessions were devoted to an account of their courtship. At the fifth session, I was told by a flushed and delighted Margaret that they had been to bed together and had had slightly awkward, but enjoyable sex. At the sixth and final session she announced that he had proposed to her and had been accepted. They were now spending several nights a week together at her flat and doing lots of things together as a couple. A new life seemed to have opened up quite unexpectedly for Margaret and we speculated about how it could have happened when it did. (We were now back to the normal sessions of thirty minutes every four weeks.) We agreed that she must have known unconsciously that she was ready to pluck up courage to talk to a man when she asked for the six sessions on sexual identity – all she needed from me was some back up while she got on with it. I had never seen Margaret looking so happy or so feminine. I told her I thought Richard (her boy friend) was a lucky man, and I meant it. Was this the happy ending we had been waiting for? Not quite.

The course of true love could not be expected to run entirely smoothly. It soon emerged that Richard lived with his mother and had considerable problems about separating from her. When pressed on the question of when he was going to make the break and move his things to Margaret's place, he tended to flap and make a bolt for home. His attempts to make the transition from son to husband were not helped by his mother coming out with outrageous remarks like 'I never eat when you are not here.'

'I can see he is like a little boy in many ways,' said Margaret. 'But I do not mind that. I think I just have to be patient. And perhaps no other man would put up with me.' She received a good deal of support from Richard's brother and sister-in-law who were clearly pleased to see Richard with a girl-friend, and have done their best to encourage him to leave home: so far without success.

I still see Margaret for half an hour every six weeks. Mostly we just talk about the ups and downs of her relationship with Richard. Some of the old feelings of depression and apprehension are still around, but Richard is a considerable antidote. They have now been together for nearly two years and I think (and hope) that they will eventually sort out their problems and move in together permanently.

4

SALLY

When a patient moves away and joins another practice, her case notes go with her. So unless I extract a few pages or keep a separate file the information is lost to me. I did keep some of Sally's original notes for a while, but when I came to look for them in my drawer, I could not find them. Probably I destroyed them as they might have embarrassed her and she certainly would not have wanted the next doctor to see them.

I last saw her about ten years ago. I remember her face and her voice very clearly but I find it hard to recall exactly what her presenting problem was. It may seem presumptuous of me to write about her at all in that case, but I think that the nature of our interaction tells more about Sally and her needs than any list of symptoms possibly could. She was a recently qualified chemist in her mid-twenties; fairly small and plump with brown curly hair and lively face. The first time she came to see me she clearly had a lot to say, and I invited her back at the end of surgery a few days later so that she could tell me the whole story. (Again, I have to say that I do not remember what it was all about).

In our first session she talked rapidly for over an hour with no sign of having finished. I invited her back for another long session and that still was not enough. So I offered her a series of six forty-five minutes sessions at weekly intervals. I felt that some sort of limit was necessary or she might go on for ever – at that stage in my career as a part-time psychotherapist I had not yet committed myself to an open-ended policy.

What was all this talk about? It was about the way no-one seemed to take enough notice of Sally or take her seriously. Her superiors at work were hurtful in this respect and so were her parents although her childhood seems to have been fairly uneventful. (She was the only child of lower middle class parents). By the time we reached the fifth session it became clear that I was not taking enough notice of her either. Why, she complained, was she being given only six sessions? Evidently that was all I thought she was worth and after that I would be glad to get rid of her. I think this was my first experience of the powerful effect of transference. Furthermore, these feelings were being expressed directly with no need for me to reveal them to the patient by interpretation. I did not need to tell her, she was telling me, that I was someone of great importance in her life from whom she demanded care and attention, and towards whom she could feel both affection and anger. Impressed and moved that she could need more of my time so desperately, I agreed to extend the sessions for a much longer period (I think I said a year). Her relief was immediate – but I was not let off the hook by any means: further challenges to my ability to give without losing control were soon forthcoming.

First of all, she told me about some counselling sessions she had had with a church minister. He had shown some interest in her problems and had agreed to take her on, as I had done, for some weekly sessions. She had become very interested in his personal life and wanted to be friendly with his wife as well. As she was a member of his congregation, this was not unreasonable, but he evidently became uneasy when Sally began telling him how jealous she felt of their married life together: especially their sex life. In accordance with the usual psychotherapeutic ground rules, he blocked questions on this subject but did not seem to be able to deflect her probing by interpreting them in terms of transference, which a more skilled practitioner might have done. The therapeutic relationship was severely strained and reached breaking point when Sally told the poor vicar that she desired him sexually and wanted to go to bed with him. I do not think she expected him to comply, but even discussing the idea with one of his parishioners in his own house was too much for him, and he hurriedly brought the counselling sessions to an end: much to Sally's disgust.

It was not long before the heat was turned on to me in the same way. She began telling me (teasingly) that there was an important question she wanted to ask me. She thought I probably would not want to answer it, but she was prepared to go on asking until I did. The question was (taking a deep breath): had I ever masturbated?

Nowadays I know that the correct way of dealing with a question like that is to say something like: 'I wonder why you should want to know that and why it is so important to you . . .' At the time I felt somewhat rattled and intruded on, and did not have this professional response to hand. I wanted to get out of the corner quickly without letting her down like the minister, so I just said, 'Yes, of course I have, just like most people.'

Again her relief at getting a straight answer was noticeable. She went on to tell me about her own masturbation and the sexual fantasies which went with it. She had had a few boyfriends and a little sexual experience but there was no-one special at the time. Sexuality seemed to obsess her and it was not something she could talk about with her parents.

As I wrote that sentence I suddenly remembered a large chunk of her past which, for some reason, I had censored out, until it was recalled by the phrase 'talk about with her parents'. Now I remember that she had become pregnant when she was about eighteen. Abortions were not readily available in those days (before the 1967 Abortion Act) and Sally had been sent to one of those 'homes for the unmarried mother and her child', which now seem totally to have disappeared. She had endured a good deal of shame and hushing up of her disgraced state and then gone through a long and painful labour. The baby (a boy) had been taken away for adoption fairly quickly (days? weeks? I have forgotten. Sally would reproach me again for not finding her important enough to remember the details.)

She seems to have received little in the way of personal support or help at the home, at least in her own perception of it, and was soon shunted back into the outside world. She must have acquired some A-levels either before or after this, and found her way to a university where she could make a fresh start.

Her parents seem to have taken the view that the whole episode was best treated as if it had never happened – they must have been very shocked and unhappy but Sally had no sympathy to spare for their feelings. She still felt a yearning to see her son again and speculated about what sort of life he was living. She soon lost touch with the baby's father and had no warm feelings left for him. Subsequent boyfriends had been unremarkable. But now her erotic feelings had a new object to focus on: me. She would introduce the subject by way of her dreams which I encouraged her to bring along in accordance with psychoanalytic practice. Her dream theatre increasingly featured scenes in which we were naked together or making love in various ways. Sometimes I would be the object of sadistic attacks in which, for example, she would take a sharp knife and carefully bisect my naked body. Sexual desire for me occupied her waking thoughts too. We had an unusually hot summer in the second year of her therapy and I started wearing tee shirts at the surgery instead of a jacket and tie. Sally would run her tongue over her lips and tell me exactly what she would like to do after removing my tee shirt – then accuse me of wearing it deliberately to provoke and frustrate her.

How did I respond to all these erotic attacks? I felt as though I was having a very bumpy ride on some sort of vehicle or possibly a wild horse and was hanging on tightly, trying to stay in control without being either carried away or thrown off. It was, of course, very flattering (and arousing) to be talked to in this way. One of my options was to succumb and let myself be physically seduced. My personal and professional responsibilities (and the corresponding sanctions to be expected from wife and disciplinary body) prevented me from making this unwise choice. It may not have been what Sally really wanted and would certainly have done neither of us any good.

My second option would have been to jump for safety before the ride got too wild and dangerous: like my predecessor, the minister, I could have ended the sessions or at least refused to listen to this sensational and provocative material. What I actually did was to listen and accept all the erotic feelings without either reciprocating them or rejecting my ardent admirer. She was aware that, among other things, she was tempting me into dangerous territory because I remember her saying that she felt pleased that I cared about her sufficiently 'to risk being struck off by the GMC' – although she did not really want that to happen. I tried to interpret her outpourings in terms of her childhood feelings about her parents, in the best psychoanalytic tradition: but, on the whole, she was much more interested in me than my interpretations. I think what really helped her was the fact that I stayed with her and let her say all these outrageous things without letting go of her, and without forgetting what she had been through – and how despairing she must often have felt underneath all the sexual bravado.

Gradually, as the weather became cooler the erotic intensity waned and our discussions became calmer. Sally acquired a boyfriend (to my relief), and began to go to bed with him with pleasure and without an unwanted pregnancy. Like a good GP I had made sure she was taking the contraceptive pill. We began to talk less about sex and more about life in general. We talked about some of her difficulties with her colleagues at work, about her relationship with her parents and about her future plans. In return for my interpretations she tried to interest me in a few of her ideas. I remember that she gave me two books to read in the course of our time together. One was a commentary on the Book of Job by C G Jung (perhaps a tribute to my patience) and the other was a book called *The Origin of Love and Hate* by Ian Suttie. I discovered that Suttie had been a psychoanalytic heretic who had broken away from Freudian doctrine because he could not accept the idea of a death instinct. His book is an argument against the necessity of there being any such unpleasant thing in the world as primary evil. Anger and hatred, when they do occur should always be seen, in his view, as the result of the love instinct frustrated. Given the opportunity, he says, love will always win through. I dismissed Suttie's argument at the time, because I thought he was wrong, and I needed to feel sure that there was only one theory I believed in. Challenges to that theory felt dangerously subversive and had to be beaten off.

Nowadays I would not be so worried. I would be more interested in what Sally was trying to tell me. Perhaps she was trying to tell us both that there was nothing evil about her: just frustrated feelings of love that needed to be understood and acknowledged. I did not return her passion (if that is really what it was), but I did care about Sally and felt affection for her. She had a good sense of humour and could always see the funny side of her amorous assaults on my professional virtue, even when she was angry at the same time. She attacked, I defended, we both got angry at times but we also enjoyed each other's company.

After two years we agreed to reduce the sessions to once a month. She was apprehensive at first, but in the event, she managed the reduction without any difficulty. Her need for me was already lessening; she had her boyfriend and her career to occupy her attention and the monthly sessions were mainly progress reports. She became engaged and then married, and at the end of another year, they moved out of the area to take up new jobs. I have not seen or heard from Sally since then, but I often wonder how she is getting on.

5

HELEN

Helen was not my patient to begin with. Probably she never wanted to be my patient at all. Her actual doctor was K, a young woman doctor from Iceland, who spent a year in the practice as a trainee. K and I had a weekly tutorial in which we would discuss, among other things, any patients who were causing her difficulty or concern. This was how I first heard about Helen. She was a twenty-one-year-old girl who was initially brought to see K by her mother because she would not eat and she had stopped going to college. She vomited frequently and had lost a stone in weight, having been fairly thin to begin with.

Mother thought that she must have some sort of organic illness which needed hospital investigation: but it did not take K very long to discover that Helen's eating problems were psychological in origin. Instead of sending her to hospital she began seeing her regularly to discuss her problems – an approach which I encouraged and supported, but without any direct involvement. It soon emerged that Helen's family was in a state of active fragmentation. Her parents were in the process of divorcing, but were still sharing the marital home. Helen's two younger brothers seemed to be in the father's camp (they eventually went with him when he moved out) while Helen took her mother's side and was even sleeping in her mother's bed while her father occupied her room.

In the course of the next few weeks, and with K's help, Helen began to eat properly again but she remained obviously depressed and withdrawn. Her mother now agreed that she was emotionally disturbed and began pressing for a psychiatric opinion. Helen was eventually admitted to the local psychiatric unit for three weeks during which K visited her twice a week and continued their therapeutic dialogue with the approval of the consultant.

Gradually Helen improved, and soon after her discharge she was able to go back to college. She continued to see K once a week and I felt pleased with both the patient's progress and my pupil's good work. I heard a good deal about Helen from K in our tutorials, but I only saw her myself when K was on holiday or for other reasons, was away from the practice. When this happened, Helen would usually have some sort of relapse (signalled by news from her mother that she was again staying at home and refusing to eat.) Mother would request me to visit her at home and Helen and I would have an awkward one-sided conversation in which her silence forced me to ask too many questions. As soon as K returned, Helen would make a miraculous recovery and I would no longer be needed. While I was relieved to see Helen recover, I could not help feeling rather excluded. It was clear that her sullen silence with me was replaced by a happy chatter as soon as she was with K again. I remembered the way the family had split along the gender boundary, with the men detached and eventually removed. It seemed to me that I was just another tiresome, unwanted male and there was nothing I could do to improve my position.

Then there was a tragedy. K's five-year-old son was knocked down and killed by a car. K was naturally devastated by the loss and went back to her home country where she stayed with her husband for six weeks until they could both recover the strength to return to their work in England. But three weeks after K's departure there was another tragedy. Helen's best friend at college, a girl called Clare, committed suicide by taking an overdose of sleeping tablets. Once again I was summoned to the house by Helen's mother.

This time poor Helen was tearful and quite eager to talk. She had spoken to Clare on the telephone, probably a few hours before she had swallowed the pills, and she reproached herself bitterly for not having realised that her friend was feeling suicidal.

'The only thing I want now is to go and join her,' she sobbed; and I shared her mother's fear that she might do it. I arranged for a home visit by a consultant psychiatrist, who said that she ought to be admitted to hospital compulsorily under the Mental Health Act if she refused to come in voluntarily.

Helen refused to have anything further to do with him or his hospital and her mother did not like the sound of the Mental Health Act either. In the end we all agreed that Helen would remain at home under her mother's close supervision and that I would keep a careful eye on her as well. In this way, we managed to keep Helen alive, eating a little, staying at home and grieving for her dead friend. A few weeks later, K returned, still grieving herself over her even more serious loss; patient and doctor were reunited.

Once again, I retired from the front line, and received reports that Helen was gradually picking up. The problem now was to get her out of the house and back to college without her mother being terrified that she would take her own life as soon as she was no longer under surveillance.

Between May and August of that year, there were several more short periods when K was away and Helen again began talking about suicide. On one occasion I was told that she had spent an entire week in bed eating nothing and talking constantly about death. But the following day, K returned from study leave, Helen bounced out of bed to keep an appointment with her and, when I looked for K after the morning surgery, I found that the pair of them had gone off to the pub for lunch. I felt very put out, and was considering taking K to task for blurring the professional boundaries by socialising with a patient. Fortunately, I recognised that the urge to deliver this reprimand came from my own feelings of exclusion – and was better set aside. Shortly after that, K's trainee year came to an end and we discussed what was to be done about Helen when K returned home. Helen agreed to come for a weekly session with me on a Monday evening. I was relieved that she had accepted me but felt apprehensive about whether I would be an adequate substitute for the doctor she really wanted.

THE WEEKLY SESSIONS

In the first session we started off on safe, neutral ground by talking about whether she should apply for a place at a hostel instead of living at home with her mother. She had discussed this with K too, and I noticed that in spite of their friendship Helen always referred to K very respectfully as 'Doctor F'. 'I just could not call her by her first name, even though she asked me to. It did not seem right.' She then said that she had not kept her appointment with the hospital psychiatrist because she did not like him. He had tried to prevent her from seeing K (Dr F), did not want Dr F to visit her in hospital and disapproved of her invitation to Helen to come and visit her in Iceland for a holiday.

The psychiatrist had clearly worried about profess-ional boundaries too – or was he just feeling the effect of Helen's powerful wish to exclude other people (especially men) from her private relationship with Dr F? I suggested, in psychoanalytic fashion, that there was a parallel with Helen's early childhood relationship with her mother. Perhaps her father always seemed to be interfering and trying to take her mother away from her. She did not reject this interpretation and seemed to find it quite interesting; at least we were having a conversation and I was not being rejected. I felt bold enough to suggest that it was always a man who tried to separate her from a nice helpful mother-person; and that she felt that I was the interfering man who was trying to take Dr F away from her at the end of their sessions. Helen said,

'Yes, you used to buzz her on the internal telephone and ask if she had finished and she would say, "just another ten minutes".'

In the next session she told me about her friendship with Clare, the girl who had killed herself.

'We were always together; we told each other everything.' Clare had been married, but a few months before her death, she had had an extramarital affair with a man called Jake. She had become pregnant as a result and her husband, realising the child would not be his own, 'forced her' to have an abortion. She had really wanted to leave her husband after that, but, according to Helen, 'She had not got the strength.'

I asked Helen what she thought of the seductive Jake and was surprised by the strength of her reaction. Her eyes blazed briefly and she said,

'He is still alive, but I want him dead. He is evil. He murdered my little Clare.' She went on to tell me that Jake was not really human, he was a kind of demon. He would enjoy the thought that he had made Helen ill as well as driving Clare to suicide. This all began to sound rather overheated. I began to get anxious about Helen's own murderous feelings, and found myself talking about the need to neutralise them by understanding what they were about and preventing them from doing harm.

I must have made quite a long speech, because when I had finished, I said I felt as though I had just preached a sermon like a minister. Helen found that quite amusing and we parted on good terms. At this stage (at every stage) I felt that our relationship was quite fragile and that I could easily lose her if I offended her in some way. Often, I had the impression that she only came out of obedience to her mother or perhaps because she knew that K wanted her to.

The following session took place on Clare's birthday. Helen said that there was no record of her name in the Book of Remembrance at the crematorium. Her ashes had just been scattered, she had been blown away as if she had never existed. Everyone except Helen wanted to forget her. When she went back to college she wanted to have 'Clare's space' in the Art room and she hoped that her tutor would permit this. I was pleased at the thought of her going back to college as the alternative plan seemed to be to commit suicide and enter 'Clare's space' that way. She was quite open about her suicidal feelings and must have been aware of the anxiety they produced in me.

In that session she also talked about her dentist who was a friendly woman and had fitted in an appointment for Helen by cancelling the appointment of another patient (a man).

'It is the second time she has done that to him – he always gets keyed up and then the appointment is cancelled.' She said she felt sorry about this but she also found it amusing. I suspect that she found it amusing to get me keyed up for nothing in a similar way.

The following week I saw her at home, but I cannot remember why. She told me about an occasion when she herself had taken an overdose. She had stopped swallowing the tablets after a while because she felt frightened. What would it be like to be dead? Did Clare know she was dead? She should have been allowed back to college for an extra year, but the tutor said it was not possible.

'He never really understood her. He could have fixed it if he had wanted to.' I immediately thought of K, whose stay in the practice had finished at the end of a year. It must have seemed to Helen that, if I had wanted to, I could have 'fixed it' for her to stay another year. There was always a man who came and spoiled everything. On my way out I noticed that the front door was kept locked and bolted.

'That is in case my father comes,' said Helen.

On my way back to the surgery, I wondered what my role was in Helen's world. Part of her seemed interested in staying alive and talking to me. Another part was still dreaming of death.

The next week I was pleased to hear that she had restarted college and that the tutor had reserved Clare's space for her. She was going to buy a book and present it to the college library in memory of Clare. She told me Clare had really loved her husband:

'She told me in a letter.' Helen seemed quite surprised at the idea, but wanted to convince me that it was true, despite the fact that she had killed herself. I told her that I

61

knew she was still thinking about death herself, and probably hoarding some sleeping tablets for another overdose. I said if she did get the urge to take them I hoped she would discuss it with me first. There was no reaction.

She continued going to college and came to see me punctually every Monday evening. She seemed to get used to this pattern and we both gradually became more relaxed. She talked a great deal about death but I felt it was better to have the subject out in the open. Once she asked me what post mortems were like. Did they put the organs back afterwards? Clare's husband had been to look at her body before the cremation. The undertaker said she would look nice but she did not, she looked horrible. I thought that death was now beginning to seem cold and horrible – not so romantic and attractive.

She started making a box for her painting materials at college. When it was finished, everyone, including the teachers, came to look at it. It was three feet long and shaped like a coffin. I said it was a child-sized coffin and she was putting her dead child self in it. We both thought about Dr F's dead little boy, and Helen talked about Dr F visiting his grave and looking at the memorial stone. But Clare had no memorial. I suggested that Helen might be wondering whether her father would forget her, now the divorce of her parents was final. She said coldly, 'I have no father.' I said I thought she needed a father as well as a mother. I could not be an actual parent to her, but could try, in the sessions to give her something of the experience of a child being cared for. This was clearly the wrong thing to say as it sank like a stone into the silence that followed.

But she continued coming on Monday evenings. Sometimes she talked freely with a child-like animation;

on other occasions she looked sulkily down at her hands and had to be prodded to make her say anything at all. Again I would find myself preaching little homilies about the need for parental care and affection; or the need to hang on to life and not give way to death.

One day she talked about applying for a course at another college.

'Where they make you concentrate really hard.' I said she did not always concentrate very hard on the work in my 'course'. Helen smiled mischievously and said,

'It is like the Child Guidance Clinic – if she did not let me play with the dolls' house, I would not talk to her!'

In the next session she reported that she had seen someone at college who looked like Jake. She shocked me a little by saying venomously that she still wanted to kill him. She had dreams in which he was lying dead at her feet. How long would they put her away for? He could not be allowed to get away with it. He had ruined Clare's relationship with her husband by seducing her, making her unfaithful and guilty.

I speculated (psychoanalytically) that Helen had an Evil-Jake part of herself which wanted to ruin the relationship between her mother and father and split them up. She said they had only stayed together for her sake and should have separated long ago. A little later she told me that her tutor had given up being anyone's personal tutor. The strain of having both Helen and Clare to cope with last year had been too much for him. He was not well. He had troubles of his own. Helen said she felt a bit responsible. Unable to resist the analyst's opening this provided, I said she was also talking about me, and wondering if I could cope with Helen without becoming ill. This did not go down well. She told me rather primly that she would 'prefer me not to talk about what we were talking about and why.' To rub it in she added that she was missing Dr F and hoped to see her when she visited England again in a few months' time. I felt suitably squashed and attempted no further transference interpretations that day.

The following week she sat down and remained silent for about fifteen minutes. Then she told me she was painting a triptych. There was a thin panel in the middle ('that is me') and a large one on either side. It was autobiographical. Yes, the two large panels could be her mother and father, but she was not thinking about her father at all nowadays.

Later on, we talked about the night Clare died. Helen had telephoned her in the morning but she was crying too much to talk. Helen rang again but the callbox machine would not accept her money. She had a feeling that Clare might have taken an overdose and she wondered whether to ring for an ambulance anyway. But did not. She told me that she and Clare had once agreed that one day they would both take an overdose and 'go together'.

I noted that Clare had now gone, but Helen had managed to stay alive. Of course I knew (I went on rashly) that she wanted to kill Evil-Jake first and then go, but she had not done so. Some part of her wanted to stay alive, was interested in life.

'And although both you and Clare wanted to die,' I said, 'you would have stopped her if you had got to her in time. You wanted to keep her alive. I want to keep you alive. Do you not think you are worth keeping?'

Helen said 'No' in a very small voice, and began to cry, just a little. I said that Dr F and I had spent a lot of time with her and talking about her. We both wanted her to live. She dried her eyes. I wondered if I was going too far, letting my own feelings disrupt her frail equilibrium.

I had to cancel the next session because of flu, and I telephoned Helen to let her know. There was a gratifying concern about my health. In the next few sessions she talked about the thesis she was writing for her degree, which her tutor had said was first class. She had also acquired a new boyfriend. Her parents were now divorced but her father was refusing to make a settlement. Helen and her mother were both changing their surnames: as if to wipe out all trace of him.

We continued weekly sessions until Christmas, when we agreed to have a four week break. When she came back in January, the first session was difficult and full of long silences. But the following week, she was very chatty, as if to make up for her coldness the week before. She seemed to be enjoying life at college, but still thought a lot about Clare. The tutor had said that he would not talk to her until he found out whether she was going to sink or swim. 'He has decided I am swimming.'

So far so good. Was it time for me to withdraw from the scene? I did not think she would miss me despite the theoretical reasons for thinking that she should. Nevertheless, I thought that the anniversary of Clare's death would be a dangerous time for her and I had better stick around until then. We agreed to go on meeting weekly till the end of March, and then reduce the sessions to once a month until Helen wanted to stop.

In the next few weeks the main theme seemed to be making fun of psychoanalysis. Dr F had sent her a book of cartoons about Freud which was hilarious. Helen said,

'It is so funny, when I am silent and you ask me what I am thinking about: it could just be what I am going to have for dinner!' But then she told me about a film she had seen in which a young man had been saved from suicide by the love of a woman of eighty. Maybe old

Freud had something worth saying after all, I thought, but kept it to myself.

The following week she again told me firmly that psychotherapy was a joke. I was no help, she said, if I behaved like a hospital psychiatrist, and that included trying to interpret what she said. But she did admit that it was helpful just to come and talk – or stay silent, if that was the way she felt. Clare had been having therapy last year, but she was 'put down to once a month', which she did not like. 'Various things were tried,' (including hypnosis) and then the therapy had been abruptly discontinued. I promised that this would never happen to Helen – she need not 'go down' to once a month if she did not want to. But she was quite content to see me a bit less often.

Late in March we had a session in which she reverted to talking about Evil-Jake.

'He will get away with it if I do not stop him.' I said I might have to try and stop her as well.

'By putting me away again?' she asked, flashing me a contemptuous look. I said no, I would not do that, I would try to persuade her not to destroy herself. I said sometimes she talked as if Jake was in her.

'He is in me.' I compared her plight to the Dracula story, in which the heroine is dying of 'anaemia', getting paler and weaker each day. The doctors do not know how to explain it – until the arrival of someone who knows what is going on and how to deal with it. Did that make any sense?

'They are always too late,' said Helen with finality.

Five days later, we met again. This was a Saturday, but I had asked her to come because it was March 29th, the anniversary of Clare's death. But I had missed the 'real' anniversary which, as far as Helen was concerned, was the previous Wednesday – because Clare had died on the

Wednesday. She had spent the day shaking, weeping and feeling suicidal, rejecting my attempt to be available to comfort her. Still, she survived; she did not kill herself.

After that we seemed to have fortnightly sessions – partly, I think, because Helen's mother wanted me to keep an eye on her more frequently. These sessions were fairly silent ones, but I contented myself with being present in the silence. In May I took my family for a holiday in Iceland where we spent a week with K and her family. Helen was naturally very interested and when I came back we spent a session watching some home movie film which I had taken there. We both found this preferable to the uncomfortable silence.

I think by this stage Helen had decided to put all the painful feelings away and try to forget about them. She really did not want me stirring them up again.

In July she invited me to her college open day. I went along and she seemed pleased to see me, relieved that I had stopped being an intense therapist, pressurising her to think about her psychic pain. She took her final examinations and was awarded a lower second class degree with which she was a little disappointed. She had no immediate career plans, but thought she would like to go into design. There seemed to be a tacit agreement that the psychotherapy sessions were over, and that if I would leave her alone, Helen would behave normally, not talk about suicide and not be a worry to her mother.

Nevertheless, I did see quite a lot of her in the year that followed. She came to the surgery as an ordinary patient, complaining of stabbing pains in the chest and palpitations. She described them as heart pains, but when I said they might come from her emotional heart rather than the hollow muscle which pumps blood round the body, she would have none of it. This was a physical heart pain, she had been having it since she was six and could she please see a cardiologist? Bowing to the inevitable, I referred her to a cardiologist who did various investigations and discovered a minor abnormality of the heart's electrical conducting system which sometime causes a rapid heart rate and enjoys the resounding name of the Wolff-Parkinson-White Syndrome. Unfortunately, this impressive diagnosis was not followed by a cure. Various tablets were tried but the pains only got worse and began to occur almost daily.

Finally the heart specialist decided that the pains which had always been atypical were not really heart pains at all; he referred her to the hospital's department of psychological medicine. Helen had an amicable chat with the psychiatrist but declined his offer of further psychotherapy.

I made one or two attempts to relate heartache to grieving for Clare, but Helen shook her head obstinately, bit back the tears, and refused to listen. Eventually the heart pains subsided on a tiny token dose of a heart tablet. They were replaced by nose bleeds and then an ingrowing toenail. In the next two years I saw her about once every two months with a succession of further physical problems, sore throats, wisdom teeth, skin rashes, coughs and colds. Then there were two cosmetic nose operations: the result of the first was unsatisfactory ('I look like a pig'), but the second was much better.

Perhaps I probed at the old psychic tender places a little too often, because she finally deserted me, four years after the therapy finished, and started taking her rather frequent physical symptoms to one of my female partners. Since then I have not seen Helen, but I have looked through her medical record, which is unexciting. She comes to the doctor about once in eight weeks with some minor symptom or other: a sore throat or a

68

migraine or indigestion.

She now has her own flat but comes back to stay with her mother at weekends. I am unclear about what she does for a living. When I see her name in the appointment book (the appointment is not, of course, to see me), I still feel a slight pang of exclusion. Perhaps I was needed in the year after Clare's death to prevent Helen from committing suicide as well. She is not going to do that now, but she wants to keep her emotional problems tightly sealed away. They leak out now and then in the form of heart pains, or headaches: but when that happens she will take them to a woman doctor and not an interfering man.

6

LOUISE

Louise was just recovering from a mystery illness when she first came to my surgery. She was a tall slightly overweight girl of twenty-four who had a bright intelligence, a confident manner and an executive job. She told me that after a holiday in France in the summer, she had developed diarrhoea and sickness which had persisted into the autumn, making her feel tired and depressed. She had been admitted to hospital for a week while various tests were done and the results of these would be sent to me together with the hospital physician's recommendations. It all seemed very business-like, with Louise in charge of the consultation, telling me what I needed to know and what I must eventually do.

When the letter from the hospital came, it proved to be rather inconclusive, but by this time Louise was feeling better. She said she had had a bad year with financial worries, and probably her illness had been largely due to 'nerves.' She was having to support her mother and had also lent some money, which she could ill afford, to her brother. Some kind of trust fund from which she had received money after her father's death had recently dried up and things were a little dodgy. She was having to work very hard.

'Not sure if I like my job or hate it,' she added, but would not be drawn any further. The next item on her agenda was a prescription for the contraceptive pill.

This request caused problems for me because there were at least three reasons why the 'pill' might not be good for her – she had a slightly raised blood pressure, she was overweight and she smoked ten cigarettes a day. Louise persuaded me to let her have the prescription in return for a promise to cut the cigarettes down and go on a reducing diet. I also offered to monitor her weight every few weeks and so we had a succession of low key meetings which enabled us to get to know each other.

Then, one day, she came along for a weight check looking tense and unhappy. She had been feeling restless, anxious, sometimes even panicky for no obvious reason. I offered her a long interview to look into the possible causes of her anxiety – and that was when I really started to find out about her history. When she was five, her father had developed serious heart disease. For the next two years he was chronically ill with frequent hospital admissions and several heart valve operations. Louise was never allowed to visit him in hospital, and when he died (she was seven) she and her elder brother were not allowed to go to the funeral. Immediately after her husband's death, her mother had 'a nervous breakdown' and was in hospital herself for many months.

Louise and her brother were sent to live with a succession of relatives, none of whom was memorable. There seems to have been a family conspiracy not to mention Father after his death and there was no opportunity for the children to mourn him properly. Now Louise says that she had a father until she was seven but she has no memory at all of what he was like.

However, in her teens, whenever someone said to her, 'Aren't you John Woodford's daughter?' she was overcome with a terrible feeling of grief and had to flee in tears.

She did well at school and went to university where she did a degree in business studies. During her three years at university she had a love affair with one of her lecturers who was a married man ten years older than herself. The affair ended when she left college and she told me,

'I got myself over it. I have no regrets. It was a good experience.' She had gone on to do a number of jobs in industry, rising quite rapidly through the echelons of junior and middle management. Soon she intended to start her own company.

'Everyone regards me as very competent,' she told me, smiling her broad, confident smile. 'I thought I could cope with anything until this illness happened.'

My impression was that when Louise lost, in effect, both her parents at the age of seven, her world had nearly caved in. But she had used her strength and courage to build up a powerful internal support system. Like an isolated house with its own electrical generator she had become independent of outside powerlines. She had made sure that she would never again have to depend on grown ups for support and comfort. Louise would be self-contained and she would climb to the top of the business world unaided.

In the circumstances, it was not really surprising that she was reluctant to accept too much help from me. When I suggested coming back for a series of sessions to talk about herself, she said,

'Do you really think it is necessary? I am feeling a lot better now.' In the end she agreed to come for six sessions, after which a holiday abroad would provide a convenient opportunity to escape. At first, she used the sessions to complain about problems at work and with her friends. Colleagues at work seemed to be taking advantage of her by taking the credit for ideas which she had given them. The boss, although very impressed with her at first, now seemed unwilling to promote her to a post with more responsibility.

Previously, she had been the one who listened to all her friends' troubles and told them what they should do; now she seemed to have cut herself off and did not want to see them anymore. She wanted to sort herself out and not be dependent on anyone. I suggested that she might be afraid of becoming dependent on me, and tried to link this with the lack of any 'dependable' parents since she was seven.

She was interested but not altogether convinced. She did not really miss her father. She wished he was still alive, but only so that he could take care of her mother and relieve Louise of the responsibility. It was true that she felt attracted to older men and had a number of affairs with married men. She did not think much about their wives, although friends sometimes told her that she was being irresponsible. After telling me this, she again referred to the occasions when someone called her 'John Woodford's daughter', and she would have to run away to hide her tears.

At the beginning of the next session, she confessed that she had nearly run away from me while she was in the waiting room.

'I want to be better now,' she said, 'I cannot stand any more of being helpless and unable to solve my own problems.' Tears ran down her cheeks for the rest of the interview. We talked about children and parents and how Louise had had to grow up too quickly. I said she need not feel ashamed of needing help from me.

'Does needing help go on for ever?' she asked, smiling

through the tears.

The following week she said she felt much better. There were no tears and she talked mainly about not being taken seriously enough at work. She had to fight for recognition but she disliked the sight of other people also striving to get more attention.

The week after that, she said she had decided to stop coming. Her smile seemed to be challenging me to try and make her stay. She was about to go on holiday to France, to an area which her family had been going to since she was two.

'I have been there twenty-seven times,' she said, 'I am always happy there, it is like Paradise. At least, it was until last time, when I became ill.' Usually her mother went with her, but this time she was going on her own. We talked a little about her relationship with her mother which was close but tempestuous.

'Now and then, I think: "when she dies, I shall be free".' This was upsetting, and made her cry. But despite her resolution to be free of me as well, she returned after three weeks' holiday and we continued her weekly sessions for another three months.

Usually she would start by saying she felt either good or bad. Then she would talk about a problem at work, which led on to relationships at work, including those with men to whom she felt attracted. Someone she got to know over the telephone had described her as 'a woman of mystery' – but she had found out, to her disappointment, that he was married. This enabled me to refer back to her father, the original married man in her life.

As usual, talking about her father made her feel tearful and want to run away. At my brother's suggestion (during one of our supervision sessions) I began to talk about 'the little girl in you' who still wanted to cuddle up to Daddy and got so upset when he was not there, that the

74

grown up Louise preferred to suppress her. This seemed to be a helpful way of describing what was going on. I tried to encourage her to feel safe enough to let the little girl part of her receive a bit of parental attention from me, although it might make her cry. She hated the thought that she was going to cry even though she might feel better for it. She was also very fearful of getting to like coming to see me too much.

She told me that she was grateful for the help I was giving her, but she also let me know that she did not want to be lured into a greater dependence than she could cope with. At our last session before Christmas she was feeling good and confident that she could manage both her work and her personal life.

'I do not want to cry today,' she said: so I held back on the interpretations and the conversation languished.

'Can I go now?' she asked; a bit like a schoolgirl asking to be excused. I said she could go and the session ended a little early. Shortly after that she telephoned me, thanked me once again for my help, but said she did not want to come any more.

During the next two years I saw Louise about once every three months, usually with a minor medical problem, such as a sore throat or a sprain. Then she began having discomfort with her periods and I wondered if she was anxious about a sexual relationship. She confirmed that she had a new boyfriend and that the relationship was 'ill-advised': but she was not ready to talk about it yet.

Two months later she telephoned to say that she was depressed, could not sleep and would like to come for another talk. When she came, she told me that the boyfriend was only twenty, and from a working class background. However, I was interested to hear that he had lost his father when he was three – so that despite the difference in social background, they had something important in common.

Originally she had thought: 'I will see how long it takes to make him care for me.' But now she cared a lot for him too – and her mother disapproved. I said I thought she might prefer to have someone dependent on her, rather than be aware of needing someone herself – someone who might let her down or even die. This brought us back to her father again, and the dreaded tears. I offered some more weekly sessions and Louise accepted readily. But, predictably, when she came the following week, everything was fine and she felt well enough to sort herself out. 'I will come back if I need another dose,' she promised. A few months later, her mother became ill and was found to have lung cancer. She had surgery and radiotherapy in hospital and her condition was eventually stabilised. My partner looked after Louise's mother and Louise herself had a succession of minor illnesses which brought her to see me about three or four times a year.

THE SECOND SERIES

About a year after her mother's illness began, Louise contacted me again and asked for some more sessions. Her mother was about to go to America to stay with relatives there for four months. The sessions also lasted four months, as though she could only attend to her own needs when her mother was safely in the hands of someone else. At first she told me about how she liked to be in control. At university, she felt she had to be involved in everything.

'I was popular, good tempered and never without a boyfriend, however disgusting.' Now she felt less in control and that was frightening. She even felt incompetent at work. After a few weeks she began to feel better again and 'much more confident.' I asked how her little girl self was feeling. Louise said it was good that the little girl had been allowed to come out and that she had been listened to.

'But now I can put her to bed again for a while.'

Despite this wish to retire behind her defences again, she continued to come to the sessions. We talked about her boyfriend who had now moved in with her.

'But he will have to go when my mother comes home.' She did not want to marry him because women always became overdependent on men when they married, and anyway her mother disapproved of him. I said I thought she had made a kind of decision when she was seven, never again to be dependent on anybody. For the next few sessions she was quite miserable, but somehow managed to stay with the unhappiness without running away from it. One day she told me that a friend at work had just come back from a holiday in Italy 'all brown and healthy - it is not fair, I could never do that.' For some reason, this made her crumple up and cry in quite a heartbreaking way for a few minutes.

The following week, she said, 'I felt like a completely different person when I was crying; I have never felt like that before.'

'Like that little girl?' I asked.

Louise said, 'I do not like that little girl. I want to shut her up in case she takes me over.' The week after that, she told me about three dreams. In the first one, she had to pay to go into a cinema, 'and I did not like that.'

This reminded me about something she had said about her brother having some home movie film of her father - which she had never seen and never wanted to see. In the second dream, she was involved with some

77

gangsters who were torturing her. One of them held her head under water so that she could not breathe, which was terrifying. In the third dream, she was talking to her director at work. He was helping her with a project and holding her hand. The dreams seemed to me to convey very clearly two conflicting views of the therapy with me. In one version I was taking her by the hand and trying to guide her; in the other I seemed like a sadistic gangster who was torturing her and trying to drown her in tears.

'I do not want the little girl to come out tonight,' she said. 'I want to get rid of her. I cannot look after her.'

'I could help you,' I said.

'No', said Louise, 'it is better to survive on my own.'

She came twice more, and then decided she had had enough. I saw her from time to time in the next few months with the minor illnesses which seemed to erupt whenever we were not having sessions. Her mother's illness entered its terminal phase and Louise nursed her at home very devotedly until she died. I went round to see Louise at home a few days later. She was still in a state of shock and her feelings were in turmoil, but she was pleased to see me. The next time I saw her, she was very controlled and businesslike while she sorted out her mother's affairs. I offered some bereavement sessions but she was not ready to let her 'little girl' come out again, and although she said she would consider my offer, I knew she would not come.

Then she did make another appearance about six weeks later. Everything seemed to have collapsed. She had given up her job to nurse her mother and now she wanted to go back into the business world but could not find an opening anywhere. Instead, she was working as a temporary typist because she needed the money.

'I cannot make any decisions; I need someone to take responsibility from me.'

Again, I offered some long sessions: she came four times and then decided, once more, that she would rather cope on her own. Thinking that, perhaps someone else might succeed in getting her to take the risk of being a little girl again, I offered to refer her to a psychotherapy clinic or a private therapist. But she did not want that either.

So poor Louise struggles on, short of money, doing a job which is a long way below her intellectual level, and with a lot of mourning still to do for her mother. At least she and the boyfriend are still together; two orphans comforting each other. I do not know what else I can do or could have done. I am still around if she needs me.

7

JENNIFER

I first met Jennifer when I had been in practice for only two months. She was an attractive-looking girl in her twenties with a lively manner (in spite of her complaint of feeling depressed) and she seemed to be able to confide in me quite easily, although it was our first encounter. She told me that she was having some group therapy about which she had mixed feelings. The group was too public for her to be able to talk about things that embarrassed her and she would really prefer to talk to somebody one-to-one, if only she could afford it.

I saw her several more times over the next few months. Although she had this friendly, confiding manner, which I found quite flattering, I realised that I did not have much idea about what was troubling her. She had been working as an assistant producer for one of the television companies but had given that job up (angrily) because it did not seem to be leading anywhere, and she was not sure what she wanted to do next. She had nearly married a year ago but had backed away at the last minute. She was the youngest of three children; she had her own flat, but was in regular touch with her parents who were also patients of the practice.

After a further discussion about the practicalities of

obtaining access to psychotherapy, I wrote a referral letter to an NHS supported psychotherapy clinic where, to my surprise and Jennifer's great satisfaction, she was offered individual therapy with a woman analyst, on a three times a week basis. The therapy went well and I saw Jennifer only occasionally over the next few months. Then I had a letter from her therapist asking if I would refer Jennifer to a plastic surgeon with a view to removing a large birthmark from one of her breasts. It seems that after much thought, the therapist and her colleagues had come to the conclusion that the distress that her 'deformity' was causing her could only be removed by surgery.

The surgeon took some persuading, because cosmetic operations were done on the NHS only with great reluctance at that time. Once he was convinced that the operation was justified, the surgeon went ahead and Jennifer was very pleased with the result. She told me that her lack of self-confidence had been largely associated with her 'dreadful secret' and now that her breasts were normal she felt much happier. The psychotherapy continued for the next two years and I saw her only occasionally for holiday immunisations or prescriptions for the contraceptive pill. She started a new job in personnel management and seemed to be thriving.

Although I did not see much of Jennifer herself, I had quite a lot to do with her family in those years, which had the effect of keeping her in my mind. Her father, unhappily, developed lung cancer which was found to be inoperable by the surgeons. In those days hospital doctors only rarely told cancer patients the truth about their illness, and GPs were not keen to do so either. Jennifer's mother felt sure that her husband wanted to know what was really wrong with him, but she could not face telling him herself. She asked me to visit them at home and tell her husband the full story.

I did not feel at all happy about this assignment but I did not want to let her down. When I arrived on the appointed day, still rehearsing what I was going to say (I had never done this before) she sat me down in the front room with her husband, poured us each a large brandy and then retired to the kitchen.

Michael Harrison, her husband, was a nice easy-going man whom it was a pleasure to talk with. He was not in pain, but felt rather weak and tired and realised that he was not getting any better. I did not mention the word 'cancer' but I told him there was a 'growth' on his lung which would not go away and would probably shorten his life. Naturally, he had already guessed the truth and was not really surprised. We drank our brandy and I promised to visit him again the following week. I continued visiting him for the next few months until, after a short illness with bronchopneumonia, he died at home.

After that I visited Jennifer's mother for a few weeks and continued to drink a glass of brandy in Michael's memory. Mrs Harrison suffered from rheumatoid arthritis and eventually had several joint replacement operations, so I continued to be closely involved as her family doctor. On my visits to the house I would occasionally meet Jennifer or her married elder sister and her children.

In the year following her father's death, Jennifer consulted me a few times with pains in her chest and difficulty in breathing. She thanked me for looking after her parents, but we did not make any connection between her physical symptoms and the loss of her father. Then I seemed to lose touch with her for about four years, until she turned up one day in April to tell me that she was feeling depressed and drinking a bottle of whisky a week. She had recently broken up with a boyfriend, work was no longer satisfying and she felt that her life had no meaning. I asked if she wanted to see her psychotherapist again and she said,

'Yes, but I feel ashamed about needing her again.'

When she came again the following week, she had repaired her defences a little, and felt she would prefer to manage without any more help. She was sleeping better and was less troubled about 'the man' but was still apprehensive that her depression might return. Having looked after her mother and father for the last few years, I now felt a sort of family doctor's concern and responsibility for Jennifer herself. I offered to see her regularly in the surgery for a few weeks to keep an eye on her and for some sort of low key psychotherapy. (I did not want to compete with what had been provided by her therapist and might still be available again.)

When she came the next time, I learned a lot more about her childhood. By this time I felt I knew the family fairly well and they seemed to be warm and close. It was a surprise to find that Jennifer, the youngest child, felt that 'no-one noticed me!' Her brother and sister seemed to have care-free lives and appeared to be uninterested when Jennifer tried to tell them how bad she felt. I do not remember that she was critical of her parents in that respect (perhaps I did not want to hear any criticism of my idealised patients) – she only said that they were unimpressed by her television work and did not give her much praise.

From her immediate family she turned to a cousin called Mary, who was much loved, but sadly died of leukaemia when she was twenty-three. After that Jennifer seems to have been fearful of loving anyone too much. Although she had sexual relationships with men, she had never really wanted to marry until recently. Her lover was 'a confirmed bachelor' who had also found it difficult to commit himself and had now broken off their engagement. However, he still telephoned now and then and sent her gifts.

I had a picture of Jennifer sitting alone in her flat at weekends, sipping a whisky, waiting for the telephone to ring, and planning to play hard to get when it did. She tried to keep herself busy with little jobs so that she would forget that she was sitting waiting to be wanted.

'If only I could have a good howl,' she said, touchingly, 'but I cannot.' I said I thought she was afraid to share her despairing feelings with me; she preferred to put on a brave face in the surgery and seek comfort from the whisky bottle when things were really bad at home.

'It is too ugly,' she agreed, and ran a finger over her eyelashes as though there might have been a tear there.

The following week, she was in a bright and brittle mood, telling me about all sorts of people she had spoken to at work. 'Chat, chat, chat,' was her phrase for this fragile, cheerful gossip. I tried to interrupt the 'chat, chat, chat,' to talk about the fears of loneliness underneath the surface. Jennifer said that giving way to sadness made her feel helpless, and there was a risk of getting too dependent on someone: ('must watch that.')

After that, she seemed a little calmer and did not have the same need to fill every minute of the day with little jobs or chatter. But she did feel afraid to go to bed because of recurrent dreams. In one of these she found herself 'in a Mexican prison cell, behind bars, facing a courtyard. I feel I know every brick in that courtyard and I have been condemned to be executed the next day: the family and the priest come to say goodbye.'

I said it reminded me of a child imprisoned behind the

84

bars of a cot, feeling condemned to solitude as the departing parents wave goodbye, and recede into the distance. Somehow this led her on to talk about a girlfriend whose boyfriend and she had been 'insepar-able': until she suddenly received a letter telling her that it was all over.

'Men can do that,' said Jennifer, 'but a woman cannot.' It was tempting to make a transference interpretation suggesting that she was afraid that I would suddenly decide to terminate her sessions, just when she was learning to let herself feel dependent; but at the time I felt it would be unwise to try and compete with her 'real' therapist, who, being a woman, was obviously much more reliable.

While I was thinking about this, I heard Jennifer say that she thought about me during the rest of the week and remembered what I had said about trying to stay with the feeling of emptiness instead of getting rid of it. I said I thought she felt she could never expect anyone to be available to comfort her.

'That feels right.'

The following week she referred to a television programme about the sudden disappearance of ships in the Bermuda triangle.

'Very frightening. Probably what will happen to me: I will just disappear and leave no mark.' I said I thought it was part of my job to keep her in my mind so she would not disappear. She needed to feel that there was someone to think about her, even worry about her.

'I do not like to think of anyone worrying about me,' said Jennifer. 'I expect people to say, "You will get over that, you will be all right, you will survive".' We agreed to have a break over Christmas, during which she would survive but I would worry about her.

In January she came back looking quite well. She told

me she had dreamed about her ex-fiancé who telephoned to say,

'The affair is dead, but we are still friends,' She had been surprised to find she could still feel regretful and sad about the end of that affair. Not to have got over it completely left her feeling vulnerable. I wanted her to be able to share her feelings of loss and loneliness with me a bit more, but she remained reluctant.

'You have not seen me at my worst – drinking and so forth. I am really not very nice.'

'Why have I not seen you like that?'

'I prefer to wait until I am a good deal more presentable before I let you see me.' She added that when she felt really bad she did not want anyone who had not also experienced the same thing to know about it. That made me feel rather disabled as her therapist: I was someone who had not suffered enough to be able to understand. However, she did subsequently refer to something I had said in that session as having 'gone in both ears.' It was something about her being able to experience an emotional jolt (like dreaming of the boyfriend) without disintegrating.

She thanked me for that and for my help generally, but she was now ready to disengage from our tentative relationship. We met a few more times at monthly intervals after which we made no further appointments – but I said she could always come back if she wanted.

Since then I have seen her only occasionally. She has a much more interesting job and seems generally happy – apart from having no 'meaningful relationship.' When I see her mother, I always ask for news of Jennifer.

'She is doing very well for herself,' says her mother, 'but it is a pity she never found anybody.'

8

ADVENTURES WITH 'THE BOYS'

When I began to look through my records and gather my
material for this book it soon became obvious that, in the
list of my psychotherapy patients, men were greatly
outnumbered by women. Indeed, there was only one
man (Duncan) with whom I had established regular
weekly sessions which continued for as long as six
months. This was puzzling and uncomfortable. Was I
guilty of blatant sex discrimination in the choice of
patients to whom I offered extended time and concern?
Was I avoiding too close a therapeutic relationship with
men because of unresolved problems of my own? Was I
getting some sort of inappropriate satisfaction from
spending a lot of time with damsels in distress, while
ignoring the equally pressing needs of my male patients?
Or could there be some more simple and reassuring
explanation?

It is well known that family doctors generally have
more consultations with women than men. This is partly
explained by biological and demographic factors. There
are many things which bring women to the surgery which
do not affect men: women need to see their doctors for
antenatal and postnatal care; they are generally the ones
who bring small children to the doctor where problems

involving both mother and child may need to be sorted out. Women see their doctors for contraceptive advice which for them is more 'medicalised'. The use of the pill and the intra-uterine coil involve medical attention in choosing the appropriate contraceptive, monitoring progress and coping with any adverse side effects. Finally, women tend to live longer than men and the average GP will have twice as many women as men over the age of seventy-five in her practice population.

Even so, when all these factors are allowed for, women still consult doctors more frequently than men and especially for psychological problems: a study by Goldberg and Huxley in 1980 showed that women were twice as likely as men to present themseves to their family doctor with a psychiatric symptom. Women seem to be more subject to depression and are more likely to be taking tranquillisers or sleeping tablets than their brothers and husbands. (Skegg et al, 1975). Why should this be so? Some writers have drawn the political conclusion that women are so exploited and ill-treated that they become neurotically ill as a result of their degraded condition. Others have observed that women are more easily able to express feelings of pain and helplessness; more able to cry and seek comfort from others. Men, by contrast, are expected to keep a stiff upper lip and suppress their emotional needs rather than appear weak and dependent. They are more likely to go to the pub and assuage their unhappiness by getting drunk than to seek help from the family doctor or psychiatrist. Some research by Mellinger and others (Mellinger, 1978) in the USA provides support for this picture.

These explanations are interesting but they did not satisfy me entirely. After all, psychotherapists do have male patients, albeit in smaller numbers. Freud wrote two major case histories about men he had treated, although it is interesting that the theory and technique of psychoanalysis grew out of his and Joseph Breuer's treatment of patients with hysteria, an illness then thought to be confined to women. In her book *One to One*, Rosemary Dinnage presents the personal accounts of therapy of twenty patients. She says that it was much more difficult to find men who were willing to talk about the experience than women: but she did manage to find eight men, whereas I could only come up with one. Where were my missing men? Had they never asked me for help, (perhaps preferring to go to my female partners), or had I brushed them aside while I concentrated on the women? Again I searched my memory and my records. Yes, there were some men who had wanted and needed more time to talk about themselves. I have clear memories of five of them but unfortunately they all belong to my early years as a GP psychotherapist and all but one have since left the practice. This means not only that I have lost touch with them but that their official records have left the practice and I do not seem to have kept any separate records of any of them, as I did with my more established psychotherapy patients. Nevertheless, I can provide a brief portrait of each of them from memory and I hope that this will throw some light on why the therapeutic relationship in each case was a brief one.

ROY

Roy was a curly-haired young man aged about nineteen. He had a variety of physical symptoms, such as nausea, headaches, and palpitations, together with an intense anxiety about his relationships with friends and people he met at work. He had a lot to talk about, but would often come at busy times when I was anxious about queues building up in the waiting room. I tried to get him to come at the end of the surgery, but he would often cancel these appointments, only to turn up again when I was harrassed and busy. He bombarded me with questions about the meaning of his symptoms and expressed irritation when I was unable to come up with a physiological explanation that satisfied him.

We did talk about his parents and his younger sister but there was no obvious problem there other than the fact that they were all desperately worried about him. I liked Roy, but I found him very frustrating; I could not satisfy his craving for explanations and cures and somehow we never settled into a rhythm of regular sessions. On one occasion he told me that he could not relax in the surgery and that he would find it easier to talk to me over a drink in the pub. So we had one session in the pub (which he appreciated) but it did not lead to any regular meetings in either pub or surgery.

At one stage he became quite seriously depressed and spent a period of several weeks in hospital. When I visited him he reproached me for not having spotted earlier how ill he was becoming. I felt quite guilty about that. On another occasion I remember him saying,

'You and I have run up quite a mileage together – why have we never succeeded in sorting out my problem?' Shortly after that he and his family moved out of the district and I have not heard from him since.

JIMMY

Jimmy had an obsessional illness. He was a cheerful, friendly man, without any affectation, I thought, although some doctors found him manipulative. He was about thirty-five when I met him; he worked in a typical obsessional's job (controlling the stocks of tiny industrial machine parts), and he lived with his wife and step-daughter in a neat, obsessional house.

Sessions with Jimmy were usually initiated by Tina, his wife, who would call me in distress when she could no longer cope with her husband's obsessional rituals. I think that he only ever came to the surgery for sickness certificates – all the real work was done in visits to his home. The call would generally come during my evening surgery and I would arrange to go round at about eight-thirty p.m., after my supper. I liked Jimmy and Tina's house because it was impeccably tidy and utterly spotless, unlike my own rather messy home. If Jimmy saw a speck on the carpet he had to clean it up at once; every item of furniture had to be properly aligned and in its place to the nearest centimetre, according to a plan which he must have had in his head.

More serious than the house tidying was the problem of morning and evening rituals. Poor Jimmy had to get up at five a.m. in order to get through all the checking of his clothes and other possessions which had to be done before he could go to work. Then, when he returned from his day's work, the checking had to be repeated in every detail. Like most obsessionals, he was painfully aware of how pointless and life-wasting all these activities were, but the inner compulsion still would not allow him to give them up. Sometimes he wept and rolled around the floor in frustration; then he would pick himself up and start checking again from the beginning.

By the time I arrived the evening checking had been done, and he was able to sit calmly in an armchair and talk to me about how it felt. Professional psycho-therapists are nowadays very wary of people with obsessional disorders and say that they respond very poorly to psychotherapy. I was probably unaware of this; besides,I know that Freud and the other early analysts had treated obsessional patients, and I wanted to help Jimmy and Tina. So we sat in their immaculate sitting room and talked about his childhood (unremarkable) and his fear that Tina would leave him if he could not stop the rituals. He very much wanted her to have his child and was delighted when she became pregnant.

Late in the pregnancy, Tina had to be admitted for rest because of high blood pressure. Jimmy became overwhelmed with misery and took an overdose so that for a few days they were both in different parts of the same hospital. Tina eventually gave birth to a little girl and when wife and daughter returned home Jimmy seemed to be able to forget his checking for a while. But a few days later he telephoned me in a state of panic to tell me he had been arrested for shoplifting.

I learned that he had desperately wanted to buy Tina a birthday present and had spent all the money he had on the gift so that there was nothing left with which to buy the groceries. Rather than make her angry he had taken a few items from a supermarket without paying for them and had instantly been spotted. He pleaded with me to appear for him in court as a character witness and I agreed (perhaps he was quite a persuasive character). On hearing the circumstances, the magistrate said he would be lenient and discharged him. Jimmy jumped up and down with joy like a delighted child to the consternation of the beak, who added hastily,

'But you are not to do it again!'

I had some fun with Jimmy. He was a nice man to be with and it was rewarding to try and help him. But the story has a sad ending. The family moved out of the area and I saw Jimmy again about a year later. Tina had left him, taking the girls with her and he was living on his own in a bed sitter. He had become seriously depressed and was on anti-depressant treatment from a hospital clinic. His obsessional rituals had vanished but he felt even worse than when he had them. A few months later I received a letter from Tina telling me that Jimmy had committed suicide.

TERRY

Terry was a drama student in his mid-twenties. He had developed a dependence on a proprietary cough mixture (containing codeine) and was drinking several bottles of it a day. Local chemists from whom he bought it could see what was going on and were becoming reluctant to supply him. But without the mixture he was unable to go on stage, learn any lines or function properly in any of his classes.

We had a few long sessions in the surgery in which I discovered that he had been separated from his mother at the age of five and only reunited with her when he was fifteen. I cannot remember anything else about his background and I no longer have his case notes, which is very frustrating. I do remember some late night telephone conversations with his tutor, who was also very worried about Terry and his future.

Terry was an engaging character, quite a charmer, and when he was not feeling anxious and oppressed by his cough mixture dependence, he had a rather infectious gaiety. On one memorable occasion, I happened to meet him in the West End of London at about three o'clock on a summer afternoon (it was my half day off). He invited me to go and have a drink with him at a club of which he was a member. The club was a small, cosy room with a bar in a basement, near Leicester Square. It seemed to be full of out of work actors, several of whom greeted Terry enthusiastically. Terry introduced me to the barman as his doctor and asked me what I would like to drink. Then he took out his wallet and discovered (in a dramatic little scene) that it was empty. This was so embarrassing, he said, but could I possibly lend him five pounds to buy the drinks with?

When we emerged, twenty minutes later, blinking in the sunshine, Terry said,

'What a lovely day! Shall we go to the park and see if we could pick up a couple of girls?' At this point, my professional instincts came belatedly to the rescue and I said that, regretfully, it was time for me to be going. Shortly after that little adventure, Terry got a job in a provincial repertory company and I have not seen him since. I wonder if he still takes the cough mixture.

MALCOLM

Malcolm was a quiet withdrawn boy of about nineteen. He was fairly short with a round face and long eyes which gave him a slightly oriental appearance. He came to the surgery initially with some physical symptoms which sounded nervous in origin. As a way of getting him to start talking about himself I asked him about his interests. He told me that he liked everything to do with soldiers and the army; weapons, uniforms, military history. He was very knowledgeable about the different regiments in the British Army.

He had applied to join the Territorial Army and was looking forward to going on some weekend camps with them. He seemed terribly shy and socially withdrawn and I wondered how he would get on with the other boy soldiers. He seemed to like talking to me and became more confident when talking about the things he knew and liked best.

I invited him to come back the following week and that led to a series of about a dozen sessions at weekly or fortnightly intervals. Then he cancelled a session and I heard nothing about Malcolm until six weeks later when his mother rang in some anxiety and told me that he was sitting at home refusing to talk to anyone. I suggested he came to see me again and after a few days he did.

This time he sat down rather stiffly and said abruptly,

'Are you Jewish?'

When I said I was, he got up and said in a flat voice, 'Is it possible to change to another doctor?' I said he could see my partner (who was not Jewish) if this was a problem, but could he tell me what the problem was? No, he could not: and he left hurriedly.

A few days later I had another call from his mother. She and her husband were desperately worried about Malcolm who would not eat anything she had cooked because he said she had been contaminated by her Jewish hairdresser. It became clear that poor Malcolm was having a schizophrenic breakdown, and he had to be admitted to hospital for treatment with anti-psychotic drugs.

I hate to think what kind of Nazi-style fantasies he had been having when he talked about those army uniforms. Perhaps he would have told me if he had not discovered that I was Jewish. Once again, my attempt to establish ongoing weekly sessions with a young man had been interrupted.

With the help of drug treatment, Malcolm's more florid delusions disappeared and he was gradually rehabilitated, being allowed home from the hospital for progressively longer periods as his mental state improved. Soon afterwards his mother died from a tragically early cerebral haemorrhage at the age of sixty. I visited Malcolm and his father at home and was pleased that he was able to greet me by name and shake hands as if we were friends, as indeed we might have been.

SIMON

Simon was the only son of rather elderly parents. I first met him when I was called to the house by his distraught mother and father because he had dropped out of college, half-way through his first term, returned home and locked himself in his bedroom. He refused to have any food and shouted,

'Leave me alone,' if his parents tried to talk to him. After calming down his mother and father, I knocked at Simon's door which was now unlocked.

He allowed me to come in and although he was taciturn at first, he gradually began to reply to some of the questions which I left hanging in the air. He told me that he had been let down by a girlfriend and since then had been unable to concentrate on his academic work. Gradually he had become more depressed and now he just wanted to be left alone until he got over it. When I observed that his parents were worried about him not eating anything, he pointed to a large bowl of fruit on the table, and said,

'Do not worry, I shall not starve.' I asked him to come to the surgery and talk to me but of course he would not. And he continued to spend all his time in bed, while his parents wrung their hands in dismay.

Mainly to show his parents I was still trying to help, I made a number of other visits in the next few days. Simon seemed quite willing to let me come in and talk to him, and at times he even became slightly animated. He dismissed psychoanalysis with scorn, but showed some interest when I told him about a book called *Oblomov* by the Russian author Goncharov. (Oblomov is a character who loses the will to get to grips with his life and stays in bed all day: to the despair of his friends.)

When I called again a few days later I saw a copy of *Oblomov* on Simon's bedside table – he had made a lightning expedition to the library to get hold of it and then hurried back to bed.

We tried having family conferences (which he would attend briefly in his dressing-gown) at which I turned my attention to the family dynamics that might be keeping the three of them locked in this unproductive situation. There was still no progress and eventually everyone's patience wore thin. His parents insisted that something must be done, and so I arranged for a consultant psychiatrist to visit him with me. I warned Simon that this was going to happen and that he might be committed to hospital if the psychiatrist felt that he was a danger to himself.

Minutes before the psychiatrist came in through the front door, Simon disappeared through the back. The psychiatrist listened to our story but pointed out that she could do nothing without a patient; she would be happy to see Simon just as soon as he turned up again. Once again I was left to comfort the parents as best I could. Happily Simon came to no harm and I had further news of him, and occasional consultations with him, from time to time. He never completed a degree course but decided to work as a gardener which he seemed to find very soothing.

He had an unsatisfactory relationship with a girl who had someone else's baby at the same time. He continued to have periods of depression during which he would retire to bed and refuse any treatment, although he seemed to get some satisfaction from the spectacle of the worried parents, girlfriends and doctors who clustered round him whenever this happened.

CONCLUSIONS

Now that I have assembled my memories of five of 'the boys', is it possible to see any patterns or common factors which might explain why, despite their need and my interest, regular weekly psychotherapy in the surgery was never properly established? At first glance all the boys seem very different; and yet I felt drawn to each of them as to a kindred spirit. Roy with his anxiety, Jimmy with his obsessions and Terry the actor were all lively and outgoing, with an ability to charm (one of the hallmarks of the psychopathic personality, I seem to remember). Malcolm, sliding gradually into schizophrenia, and Simon, holed up in his bedroom, were less accessible characters, but I think they appealed to a different side of me, more secretive and solitary.

All (except Malcolm) had a tendency to lure me out of the surgery and involve me in some kind of mild adventure on, or just over, the professional boundary: Roy got me into a pub, Terry into the actors' drinking club (but no further); while Jimmy and Simon both induced me to spend evenings at their homes long after the surgery was over. It looks as though I was content to be led (or seduced), rather than laying down my own terms. Why did I not say, 'If you want my professional help, you must come to the surgery at an appointed time and stay for exactly forty-five minutes' – as I did with Duncan and the women patients?

With Simon this would clearly have been a non-starter;

Malcolm did come regularly until his breakdown. With the others, I think I could have tried harder to establish a firm setting in the consulting room. My relationships with all the patients in this chapter happened more than ten years ago, when I was less clear about the way to proceed. Today, rather than allowing events and personalities carry me away, I am more likely to bear in mind that psychotherapy means a commitment by both doctor and patient for a number of years. I am very much aware that I can only honour such a commitment with two or three people at a time.

And yet, when all these factors are allowed for, there remains the question of gender difference, which still has not been adequately explained. In those early years, I made and honoured commitments to women patients who were willing to come to the surgery and stick to the rules. Perhaps women really are more willing to experience and re-experience those feelings of dependence and loss which are so deeply rooted in childhood. Men, on the other hand, are expected to be tough and sturdy; not to cry over their lost love, but play games, joke about their problems if possible and, if this is not possible, to be strong, silent and self-sufficient. Perhaps, as a man myself, I find the notion of a man in distress upsetting – and prefer to play games, have little adventures, and then break off. Nowadays, I notice that the troubled young men in the practice tend to confide in the trainee doctor: who is invariably receptive, patient and sympathetic – and usually feminine in gender.

9

PERSONAL ANALYSIS

In this chapter I would like to give an account of my own experience of psychotherapy as a patient. As a result of my deepening interest in psychoanalytic ideas and my increasing activity as a GP psychotherapist, I decided that it was important for me to find out for myself what psychotherapy felt like.

My interest in psychoanalysis had begun much earlier. I remember when I was about sixteen, discovering some books by Freud in my parents' bookcase, and becoming absorbed in them. I began to get other books by or about Freud from the library, and even chose a copy of the *New Introductory Lectures* as a school prize.

In my late teens, Freud's ideas seemed to provide me with a much needed key to the meaning of human thoughts, feelings and behaviour, I believed that I could explain the motives of everyone around me in Freud's terms, and this in turn made me feel much more in control of my world. Later on, at university and medical school, I came across the arguments against psycho-analysis for the first time and felt very uneasy about the way my certainty had been undermined. I also felt angry with Freud for letting me down.

I veered over to being an opponent and critic of

psychoanalysis, whose theories, I now told anyone who was interested, were incapable of proof and therefore of no scientific value. And yet Freud's ideas still had a strong pull for me; at successive stages of my life I would go back to his works and those of his followers and struggle to understand them. (They now seemed much more difficult than when I was sixteen) Enthusiasm and a wish to know more, would be followed by another wave of disillusionment and turning away from Freud.

Then, in the 1970s, I found myself offering to help troubled patients in my practice by listening to their problems and trying to make sense of them.

One of my elder brothers had plunged into psycho-analysis more wholeheartedly and was now a trained, practising analyst as well as a GP. He encouraged me to take on selected patients for individual psychotherapy and gave me supervision sessions in which he showed me how to proceed along psychoanalytic lines. (See 'Beginnings').

I knew that the analytic training involved having a personal analysis, although I was not quite sure why. The usual explanation was that it was necessary to understand and resolve your own emotional problems in case they were stirred up by those of the patient and thus interfered with the treatment. There is some truth in this, and it is a praiseworthy aim, but one wonders how far it is possible for any analyst to achieve this kind of self-awareness.

It seems to me more likely that the chief purpose of personal analysis is to teach the student the technique; having experienced it himself at first-hand, he can then apply it to his own patients. For me there seemed also to be an element of initiation, of having to go through the fire in order to be admitted to the Brotherhood. The echoes of my adolescent attraction to psychoanalysis still made me think of its practitioners as high priests who knew the secrets of the human mind: and I desperately wanted to be one of them. At the same time, my reservations about the scientific status of psychoanalysis made me hold back from committing myself to applying for training at this stage. It would also have been very expensive in both money and time. The training analysis itself usually lasts for four years, with sessions four times a week at a cost in present day prices of about £20 per session. In addition the trainee has to attend evening lectures and take on his own patient four or five times a week with weekly supervision.

I did not feel ready for such a deep involvement and had other things I wanted to do with my money and spare time. All the same, thoughts of analysis continued to preoccupy me and I wondered if there was some way in which I could sample the experience. Perhaps I could start some analysis on a once or twice a week basis to see how I found it? My brother recommended a discussion with a senior colleague for whom he had great respect, and he in turn referred me to another analyst whose work and theoretical orientation he approved of. Thus, I found myself, one morning in the autumn of 1976, pressing the doorbell of a consulting suite in a Georgian terrace in north London, and waiting to meet my analyst.

Mrs M (as I shall call her) was a woman in her mid-fifties. My first impression was that she was quite severe and uncompromising. As we discussed arrangements for appointment times and fees I began to feel like a small boy being dominated by a boarding school matron. She said I must come for sessions at least twice a week, always at the same time of day. There was no question of taking holidays except when she had hers; and all sessions would have to be paid for whether I came or not. Even though twice-a-week was only a taste, as she put it, and most patients came more often, I felt trapped and imposed on. I was not a patient after all, but more like a colleague. There was nothing wrong with me: I just wanted to find out a bit more about myself in a spirit of scientific enquiry. Or that is what I told myself, on the way home from that first meeting.

And so I reported to her every Tuesday and Friday at (or shortly after) the appointed time. I lay on the divan bed and talked about myself while Mrs M sat in the customary analyst's position at the head of the bed, out of sight, but very much present as a voice. I was surprised to find that she used her voice almost like a singer or an actress, making it loud or soft, harsh or gentle, depending on the kind of feelings she was reflecting. I gave her an outline of my life story in that first session and received in return some interpretations which I found rather confusing. I was just beginning to get the hang of it when Mrs M said,

'Well,' in a brisk tone. There was a silence and then she said, 'It is time to stop for today.' I soon realised that 'Well' was the word she used to signal the end of the session, after exactly fifty minutes (with rare exceptions). I was not supposed to say any more after that, but get up obediently from the couch, turn to say goodbye and leave the room. Sometimes the conclusion seemed hurtfully abrupt and I got some idea of what it must be like for my patients when I did something similar to them. Whatever I was about to say next simply had to wait for the following session.

What did we talk about? To start with, I gave her an account of my life story and my present situation: marriage, family, work and so forth. Then, following the traditional method, I was invited to talk about anything that came into my head: thoughts about the day's events, reminiscences brought up by free association, views, attitudes, feelings about various people in my life, dreams and fantasies.

There were some things which I found too private and personal to include in this account, and I hope the reader will forgive me for missing them out. Nevertheless, I hope that even after the censorship, enough remains to give some sort of impression of what the experience was like.

In the course of the next few months, I became very familiar with Mrs M's working hypothesis about me. She saw me as a small boy (perhaps three or four) who desperately needs love and attention from his Mummy but fears that he will be ignored because he is so small and insignificant. He wants to be liked by everyone and so is anxious to be obliging, but also gets very angry if the grown-ups ignore him or will not reveal their secrets (such as psychoanalysis).

I went along with this scenario up to a point. Many of the things she said in that first year seemed to ring true. She pointed out, for example, that I found it difficult to say no (I could not leave a bookshop without buying something), hated to be kept waiting because I found it humiliating, and preferred to write off my mistakes rather than try to repair the damage. However, there were many other suggestions about me and my thoughts which were difficult or impossible to accept as having anything to do with me. I was quite surprised at the amount of interpreting she did, as I had previously pictured the analyst's role as that of a listener who made the occasional observation, but for the most part, allowed the patient to draw conclusions for himself.

On the other hand, I was not surprised that Mrs M revealed very little about herself. I knew that, according to the classical view, the analyst was supposed to be like a polished mirror in which the patient sees only the reflection of his own feelings. The analysis is concerned only with the patient's transference feelings about her; those feelings which properly attach to his parents, or other figures of importance in his infancy. These feelings can then be interpreted and placed in their proper context.

There is supposed to be no relationship with the analyst as a person, except the rather business-like one of partnership in the 'treatment alliance'. However, many analysts and therapists have expressed discomfort with this strict line and have observed that there is a genuine feeling relationship between patient and therapist which makes a significant, perhaps crucial, contribution to the success of the therapy. For a long time, I have felt more sympathy with this point of view, and it is interesting that some of the incidents I remember best from my analysis are those when the professional mask was allowed to slip, and the 'real' Mrs M was revealed for a few illuminating moments. I think I liked the real person better than the professional analyst with her insistence on sticking to her theory-laden interpretations.

An early glimpse of my analyst as a person came when I mentioned a visit to the opera. She could not resist sharing her enthusiasm for Mozart and I remember her saying how much more sensible the women were than the men in *The Marriage of Figaro*. On another occasion, I had been rather parsimonious with my dreams, and analysts love dreams better than any other kind of material: they cannot get enough of them. I had said very little and been very remote for most of the session (one of my annoying tricks) but, ten minutes before the end, I announced that I had a dream to tell her. Mrs M exclaimed,

'Oh, I could hit you!' I still treasure that exasperated, but affectionate little outburst. As we approached the first holiday break, she began to warn me that I would miss her and be angry with her for deserting me, like an absentee parent. In fact, I was quite looking forward to a respite from the twice-weekly drive to the sessions through heavy traffic, and rejected the idea totally. However, she did surprise my feelings by adding that she might be going to miss me. She was very keen on telling me that I dealt with unwanted feelings by projecting them into her.

'If anyone is going to feel abandoned over the holiday,' she would say, 'it certainly will not be you!'

I did not feel abandoned and I continued to attend twice a week except for holidays. My attentiveness as a pupil varied considerably. On some days I would follow her explanation of my thoughts with interest; on others I woud feel bored or confused or frankly dismissive. Whenever I could feel myself as a little boy with Mrs M as my mother, things went well, but the feeling was difficult to sustain.

By the end of the summer term I was having doubts about whether I wanted to continue, particularly in view of the inconvenience and the expense. In the autumn things were better. Mrs M seemed less dogmatic and even admitted that one of her interpretations had been inaccurate. I was able to confide some embarrassing memories from my childhood and adolescence which I had never talked about to anyone. I felt that I could trust her and that she genuinely cared for me. But again, the mood did not last.

By November I was reproaching her for meeting my honest doubts and reservations with text book interpretations about resistance, rather than with real understanding. She seemed to lose patience herself, and said that our work would possibly – or probably – not succeed. I found that a rather chilling pronouncement; it made me feel like a failure.

The following week I asked if she thought it was worth going on after Christmas, and she replied that I would need at least four sessions a week to hold on to what she was able to give me. I had not realised that I would be such a difficult case although I can now see that at that stage I did not believe I had any personal (as opposed to professional) need for psychotherapy. Professionally, my thoughts were also turning to the idea of applying to the Institute of Psychoanalysis for formal training. This might involve a training analysis with a different analyst. We agreed that I would have a break for a few months while I sorted out what I wanted to do: train at the Institute, come back to Mrs M on a four-times-a-week basis, or give up altogether. We parted amicably and I wondered if I would ever see her again.

During the next six months I wrestled with the personal, professional and financial implications of training as an analyst. Gradually I reached the conclusion that I wanted above all to be an analyst, and that I was now prepared for the necessary sacrifices. While continuing to work as a GP to support myself and my family, I would have to devote my afternoons to personal analysis and then, after a year, to treating analytic patients under supervision as well. Three evenings a week would be taken up by the academic course of lectures provided by the Institute. The whole thing would last at least four years and would be so expensive that I would have to take out a large bank loan to finance it. But my brother had done it, so why not me? I sent in my application in June and was interviewed in September.

I had two interviews, each lasting nearly two hours, and both taking place on the same gruelling day. The morning interview was with a woman analyst who was friendly and with whom I felt at ease. She expressed a few

107

reservations about my ability to get in touch with my own emotions, but after fifteen months with Mrs M this was no longer a surprise. She congratulated me on the way I had managed to utilise my defences to cope effectively with life: from an analyst this is something of a backhanded compliment.

That interview took place at her home; the second one was at the Institute itself, in a dingy, poorly-lit office which looked as if it did not belong to anybody. My second interviewer was a dry, remote man who gave me the feeling that he was seeing me only to oblige his colleagues and would have preferred to be doing something else. I was anxious to hold nothing back and told him quite a lot about myself – but at the end, I felt I had entrusted it to the wrong person. He also told me that my 'symptom' was 'emotional denial,' but admitted that I had been 'very frank.' I crawled home, feeling exhausted and ill-used. I was sure I would not be accepted.

When the letter of rejection actually came, I felt even worse for a while; a failure in the thing I wanted most in the world. I discussed the position with my analyst brother who told me that the same thing had happened to him on his first application. But undeterred, he had started analysis as a humble patient, and after a second application a year or two later, he had been accepted.

Much encouraged, I decided to do the same. The only problem was that Mrs M was not a designated training analyst and time spent with her would not count towards my formal training. If I went back to her for, say, four or five years, I would still be required to have a further four years of treatment with an approved training analyst. This seemed crazy, but my brother and his senior colleague both made it clear that, in their view, an analysis with Mrs M would be of incalculable value for my personal growth and development. Whereas the official training analysis would be almost a formality; an experience from which I would emerge 'unscathed and unchanged.'

The psychoanalytic movement is, of course, riven with doctrinal differences. My brother, his colleague and Mrs M all belonged to a particular school (I almost said a sect) which believed it had a unique claim on the truth. Or at least, a better way of going about psychoanalysis than any of the others. For those with an interest in these matters, I should add that they were disciples of Melanie Klein, a British analyst who made some revolutionary modifications to Freud's ideas, which have become very influential in Britain although not in continental Europe or North America.

Mrs Klein had modernised analytic theory by drawing attention to the importance of the early mother-child relationship and substantially altered the technique by her overwhelming emphasis on interpreting the transference. That is to say, she and her followers believed in relating every utterance by the patient to the relationship between the analyst as Mother and the patient as Baby. After fifteen months with Mrs M I was quite accustomed to this style of working although I did not always care for it.

My brother's group had distanced themselves from the main body of Kleinians by their adherence to the ideas of another theoretical innovator, a Kleinian analyst called Wilfred Bion. Bion's writings employ mathematical and philosophical concepts which I find very difficult to follow. One of his important contributions which I can understand, is the idea that the infant needs to develop the capacity to think about emotional experiences in order to make sense of them. The mother's function is to act as a 'container' to receive her

109

baby's chaotic feelings and order them for her. If all goes well, the baby can gradually 'introject' this maternal function and learn to perform it for herself.

All of which is very interesting, but how much does it matter whether your analyst has incorporated the latest theoretical contributions into her technique? My advisers left me in no doubt that it mattered, because, they believed, if I understand them correctly, that these ideas had the power to change you for the better, in a way which other forms of analysis, however conscientiously carried out, were unable to match. If I went back to Mrs M I would almost certainly emerge as a better person. I was beginning to feel a nostalgic wish to return to her in any case, and did not relish the idea of starting again with someone new.

And so in January, I returned to Mrs M after an absence of exactly a year. This time I was seeing her four times a week, from Tuesday to Friday. The increased intensity undoubtedly helped us, but two other momentous events in my life also served to put me in touch with my feelings and make me aware of myself as a person who needed help. A few days before the analysis restarted, my holiday in Yorkshire was interrupted by a message from a neighbour at home telling me that a pipe in our house had burst after a heavy frost, and the house was flooded.

I left my wife and children staying with my mother and returned alone to view the damage. Half the house was ankle deep in water, carpets were sodden, ceilings had fallen in; my house seemed to be destroyed. In particular, the sight of my little son's ruined bedroom, with his drawings drooping pathetically from the damp walls, reduced me to unaccustomed tears. I was comforted by friends who gave me a dry bed to sleep in. I found a plumber and other professionals, and gradually the house was restored to normal. But the experience of having my cosy familiar home half-destroyed was quite devastating.

The second shock was even worse. On March 3rd, I was sitting in the surgery talking to K, my trainee, when she received a telephone call telling her that her five-year-old son had been knocked down and, as we later discovered, killed, by a car. I went with the poor grieving mother to the hospital and then to the mortuary to see the body of her child. Then I took her home where there were friends and neighbours to support her (her husband was out of the country) and I spent the next few days in a state of shock. The sound of the bereft mother's crying echoed constantly through my head and gave me no peace.

I was desperately sad for K and her family, but my own deeper feelings were somehow shaken loose in a way which seemed quite new. The little boy died on a Saturday and it was Tuesday before I got back to Mrs M and told her what had happened. For the first time, I cried with her, and felt some relief from the way my grief was accepted and 'contained.' I knew that she was genuinely moved and upset as well. Then she suggested, quite gently, that I had in some sense died myself as a little boy, and wanted a mother to cry over me as K had cried over her lost son. I cried quite a lot in the next few sessions and was comforted by her words (but not physically: analysts do not hold your hand however bad you feel).

For a few weeks I felt that she was a firm presence in my life, supporting me, giving me permission to cry for myself as well as for K. We also had some fun together; I made her laugh by talking in funny voices and for a while we were like a mother and baby enjoying each other's company. Then came the Easter holiday.

When we resumed the sessions again I felt under pressure to 'work' without really knowing what I was supposed to be doing. I seemed unable or unwilling to understand the language of her more detailed interpretations, which often seemed absurd and over the top. For example, when I mentioned feeling left out when K and Helen (one of our patients) went to the pub together (see 'Helen' chapter), I was told that I was really describing a fantasy about Mrs M's breasts feeding each other, instead of my infant self.

On another occasion, my pleasure in escaping the noise and traffic fumes of the city by going into a quiet and tranquil church was described as 'seeking refuge from your dirty thoughts.' 'Dirty thoughts' turned out to be revengeful feelings about bad Mummies who abandon their babies at the weekend and go to have sex with their husbands etc. The trouble with me was that I never really missed her or pined for her at the weekends or in the holidays as a patient in analysis is supposed to do. The transference never took a proper grip on me. And yet, every so often she would say something that would touch me, make me feel she cared for me and that I needed that kind of care.

She was amazingly patient in putting up with my moody silences, my sarcasm and my ridicule. I suppose her patience was rewarded and her hopes revived whenever I melted a little and allowed my infant self to emerge for a while. Then in September the infant discovered he had a rival sibling. I learned from my brother that his junior partner in general practice, a contemporary and friend of mine, had also started sessions with Mrs M. I felt absurdly jealous about this and reproached her for making me share her with another baby. I warned her to be careful not to get us mixed up in her mind but she did not appear to take my fears very seriously.

Looking back, I think that our failure to deal adequately with the issue of my sibling jealousy was an important factor in preventing me from accepting Mrs M as a transference Mummy. She might disagree, and there were other factors. But I continued to brood about my rival and my discomfort was not helped by the frequent occasions when our cars crossed on the way to and from Mrs M's consulting room: we even had consecutive appointments.

Nevertheless, the analysis continued with its usual ups and downs. Two entries from my diary illustrate the way I lurched between acceptance of Mrs M, and rejection. In late September I received a letter from K with a sad line about searching for her dead little boy and being unable to find him. In telling this to Mrs M I really felt as if I were her little boy whom she almost lost (did lose for a year). I felt that I had become a different person, more sensitive to tears and sadness and also to children. Then, in December I told her a strange dream about a uterus 'invading the whole body.' She said I was talking about her sexual intercourse with her husband arousing my jealousy and invading my whole consciousness. This took my breath away. (I had met her husband, on one occasion when I had arrived on the wrong day. He seemed a very amiable fellow of whom I was not remotely jealous). So I said, 'Balls', very rudely, to that interpretation, and Mrs M just said, 'Well', indicating that time was up anyway!

The analysis continued for another two and a half years. I could describe many more incidents both positive and negative which enlivened our relationship, but this account is in danger of becoming excessively long. In any case, the main features were laid down in the first year of four times a week and I think Mrs M might

113

agree that we made little progress after that. In the last year I became increasingly restive and began to talk about leaving. She expressed some impatience and I asked her why she bothered to continue with me. 'If only you knew,' she said, 'how often I have thought of kicking you out.'

'Why don't you, then?' I challenged.

'Because,' she said, 'there was evidence of interest and appreciation from you – but not very much.' Nevertheless, she still hoped that, one day, I might 'decide to rejoin the human race.' Bloody cheek, I thought. Am I really so cold and remote? In November I tried to make her give up, but she just said,

'You are always like this in November and December. It is a difficult time of year for you.' I warmed up a little now and then after that. But after Christmas I became convinced that we were getting nowhere. I gave notice that I would leave at Easter and when the time came we parted on good terms.

She had tried very hard to hold on to her lost little boy: I found her determination and her concern for me quite moving. Unfortunately, I think she was, to some extent, a prisoner of her technique and interpretive language. If she had been able to set them aside a little more and talk to me in a language I could understand better, I might have learned to sustain my trust in her – and allowed the lost little boy to emerge for more than a few moments at a time. Then, perhaps, in the process of having my chaotic infant feelings returned to me in an ordered form (as Bion would put it) I might have become more sane, more enriched, more in touch with my emotions, better able to live with myself and my loved ones, who knows? It did not happen and I have some regrets about that. But the experience did not leave me untouched by any means.

I did learn to free my emotions a little more and found that I was better able to share the feelings of other people, especially my patients. My work with my psychotherapy patients was also greatly influenced (rightly or wrongly) and during the period of my analysis I often found myself talking to them with her voice, saying the sort of things to them that she would say to me. I felt a little guilty about this at the time, as though I was stealing from her; but in retrospect it seems more as if I was using something that she had given me freely. Perhaps it was unfortunate that I could only use the gift on my patients and not on myself.

She did cure me of wanting to train as an analyst. It seemed to happen one day when she said,

'You know, there is nothing especially wonderful about being an analyst. It is just a job like any other. And you seem to enjoy your work as a GP, so why change?' I thought about this and said to myself, do I really want to spend another four years training to do a different kind of work, which I may not even like, just so I can call myself an analyst? Could I really cope with seeing people for four or five long sessions a week? And that was the end of my ambition to become an analyst (although I still have occasional pangs of envy when I hear an analyst saying something mysterious.)

I remain grateful to Mrs M for the time she devoted to me, for her patience, her good humour and her concern for me as a person. I think of her with affection and with respect.

10

HOW DOES PSYCHOTHERAPY WORK?

I have already described how my interest in psychotherapy began with my discovery of Freud's theories and
my delight in the way they seemed to provide a unifying
explanation for all human behaviour. Disenchantment
followed, when the theories failed to stand up to the
standards of proof which scientists expected. Later on,
my interest in Freud's ideas was reawakened as I began to
feel the need to understand and help some of my
emotionally troubled patients in general practice.
Psychoanalysis has certainly been a great help to me in
this work, but I remain ambivalent, to use a psycho-
analytical word, about how far Freud's theory, or indeed
anybody's theory, can cure or relieve human suffering.

These days I am more inclined to believe that ordinary
human qualities such as patience, steadfastness, empathy, interest, and even affection, on the part of the
therapist are of greater value in helping patients to feel
and function better. All the same, to embody these things
for a patient is to be something like a good or 'good
enough' parent; and that analogy or interpretation takes
us straight back to Freud and transference (of which
more later). So I cannot reject psychoanalysis entirely,
although I am unhappy about the rigidity with which the

ideas are often applied. And when I look at some of the literature on psychoanalytic technique I find I am in good and plentiful company.

There seem to be two quite distinct attitudes to the practice of psychotherapy, each of which has its champions and its adversaries. They might be called the Conservative and the Liberal, or the Scientific and the Humanist, the Rational and the Emotional: perhaps even the Masculine and the Feminine. For simplicity I shall refer to them as the Hard and the Soft.

The hard analyst or therapist believes totally in the truth of the theory he has learned at his training institute. Consequently he sees interpretation as all-important. His attitude to the patient tends to be distant, detached, impersonal, slightly mysterious and emotionally cold. He makes a point of revealing as little as possible of his own personality to his patient and never talks about his private life. He does not accept gifts (even at Christmas), he does not apologise even if he is in the wrong and he does not allow his hand to be held even in moments of extreme distress. If the patient wishes for any of these things, the wish will be explored and interpreted but not gratified.

The hard analyst believes that the patient needs to feel deeply about him in the transference so that the feelings can be interpreted and insight acquired. If he notices any feelings about the patient in himself, the hard analyst compartmentalises them as counter-transference phenomena – which also need to be analysed and interpreted. These feelings are in an important sense unreal, have nothing to do with him personally, (they could happen to any analyst) and need not touch him. (There is a good description of the views of the hard analyst in Janet Malcolm's book *Psychoanalysis, the Impossible Profession* (Malcolm, 1978) in which she

117

interviews a typical member of this wing of the movement.)

The soft analyst (or therapist), on the other hand, does not regard his theoretical material as divinely inspired. Although trained in one tradition, he may utilise all sorts of ideas from other traditions if they appeal to him personally and seem to be helpful. The soft analyst uses interpretation too, but more sparingly. He is much more aware of his supportive role as one human being who has taken on the responsibility of caring for another. His attitude to the patient tends to be warm, close, concerned, empathetic and natural. He does not need to conceal his own personality or personal circumstances from his patient. It is no big deal if the patient wants to know how many children he has or where he is going for his holidays. He may well accept gifts and, at times, even allow some physical contact.

Obviously these descriptions are slightly exaggerated and they apply to the extreme ends of the spectrum of psychotherapeutic attitude. Most therapists are a bit of a mixture of hard and soft and will lie somewhere in the middle of the range. Nevertheless there is still a good deal of debate and disagreement between the two wings and this conflict has been going on, often passionately, since the earliest days of psychoanalysis.

Freud himself, with his background in medicine and neurology, saw analysis as a scientific technique whose purpose was to elicit 'the truth' about human mental processes. In his view, the analyst's therapeutic function was simply to pass on the good news to the patient, overcoming the latter's resistance, sometimes easily – more often with difficulty. The patient's emotions (and any that were evoked in the analyst) were looked at and analysed with detachment and objectivity.

In a paper called *Recommendations to Physicians Practising*

Psychoanalysis (Freud, 1912) he writes 'I cannot advise my colleagues too urgently to model themselves during psychoanalytic treatment on the surgeon, who puts aside all his feelings, even his human sympathy, and concentrates his mental forces on the single aim of performing the operation as skilfully as possible.'

And yet we also know that Freud was very much aware of the importance of the emotional bond between patient and physician. At the end of his Introductory Lecture on Psychoanalysis No 27 (on transference) he says,

'What turns the scale in his (the patient's) struggle is not his intellectual insight which is neither strong enough nor free enough for such an achievement – but simply and solely his relation to the doctor.'

Unlike his older colleague and teacher, Joseph Breuer, Freud was not frightened or deterred when a female patient flung her arms round him. His discovery of the transference provided an explanation for that, and was of immense importance for psychoanalysis. At the same time I suspect that the concept of transference enabled him to distance himself from his patients' feelings by turning them into objects of scientific study. His patients' love for him and need for him were really feelings belonging to their infancy and their relations with their parents; while they stirred his scientific excitement they need not arouse him personally.

Nevertheless, we know from the personal reminiscences of some of his patients and pupils that his manner in analysis was often friendly and informal. He seems to have been willing on some occasions at least, to break most of the rules that now stand in his name. For example, according to Paul Roazen, who collected reminiscences from many people who had known Freud (Roazen, 1971) he would sometimes analyse people living as guests in his house, he would lend patients books, exchange presents with them, tell jokes, compliment a patient on her dress, recommend a specific marriage choice, or after interpreting a particular dream remark (on one occasion)

'Now you are going to get well.' (Roazen pp 140-141). Such human and unsurgical behaviour is not to be found however in his case histories or prescriptive writings on technique for others: it seems possible that he was hardly aware of this side of his analytic style, or considered it to be somehow external to the analytic process being carried out by Freud the scientist.

It is interesting that, Freud's most famous patient, Sergei Pankovski, the subject of the 'Wolf Man'case history, when interviewed in his old age was quite dismissive of Freud's elaborate interpretation of his dreams, but very appreciative of Freud's concern and kindness to him over the years (Obholzer, 1980).

Freud's pupil and colleague, Sandor Ferenczi, was a very different personality, much warmer and more open to his patients' feelings. Although he accepted Freud's ideas totally at first and was a master of the classical technique, we can see from his Clinical Diary (Ferenczi, ed Dupont, J., 1988) that towards the end of his life (1932) he was very unhappy with the coldness and lack of humanity of psychoanalysis. He noted that many of his patients had suffered at the hands of cold, remote or even brutal parents; when they came into analysis they found themselves with an analytic 'parent' who behaved in a very similar way. Ferenczi comes to the conclusion that:

'No analysis can succeed if we do not succeed in really loving the patient. Every patient has the right to be cared for as an ill-treated, unhappy child.' (p 130). Later he quotes the reproaches of a woman patient (p 199):

120

1) Psychoanalysis lures patients in 'transference'. The profound understanding and the keen interest in the most minute details of their life history . . . are naturally interpreted by the patients as a sign of profound personal friendship, indeed tenderness.

2) As most patients are psychic shipwrecks, who will clutch at any straw, they become blind and deaf to the facts that would indicate to them how little personal interest analysts have in their patients.

3) Meanwhile the patients' unconscious perceives all the negative feelings in the analyst (boredom, irritation, feelings of hate when the patient says something unpleasant or something that stirs up the doctor's complexes) . . .

He concludes:

'As a result of infantile experiences of the same kind it becomes impossible to detach oneself from him (the analyst) . . . no matter how long the unsuccessful work has been going on, just as a child cannot run away from home (because left to his own devices he feels helpless).'

Ferenczi's ideas led to a serious disagreement with Freud who, in a letter in 1931, is disturbed to hear that Ferenczi 'was kissing his patients and allowing them to kiss him as part of the motherly affection he thought patients needed' (Roazen, p 367). Perhaps Ferenczi went a little too far but nevertheless his ideas and feelings are important and he is to be respected as the first psychoanalyst to proclaim that the 'real' relationship between doctor and patient was the important factor in helping people to get well.

'Without sympathy,' says Ferenczi, 'there is no healing. (At most, insight into the genesis of the illness)'. (Ferenczi, p 200). Ernest Jones, in his biography of Freud, said that Ferenczi was mentally ill at this stage of his life and the orthodox analysts refused to take him seriously. Nevertheless, we begin to see in the writings of subsequent analysts, increasing reference to the notion that something more than the classical technique might be needed, at least in certain cases.

In the 1940s, Franz Alexander described analysis as providing a 'Corrective emotional experience' which served to make up for some of the deficiencies in the patient's childhood. He became the father of a school of 'soft' analysis in America which flourished for a while until it was overtaken by a revival of the 'hard' tradition. Meanwhile, in Britain, Melanie Klein published a number of papers which modified Freud's theory considerably and gave much more attention to the close relationship between mother and infant, and taught that this relationship was faithfully replicated in the patient-analyst relationship. However, she and her followers see the latter entirely as a transference relationship to be interpreted to the patient with complete consistency. Much as I like their ideas, I have to assign the Kleinians to the hard side of the analytic attitude spectrum.

Later on in the 1950s, Donald Winnicott, who had been much influenced by Melanie Klein, began to talk about the analyst providing mothering as well as interpretation of mother-seeking feelings. However, he was very careful to say that this sort of analytic function could only apply in borderline patients who were so severely disturbed that they could not recognise interpretations and were thus unable to respond to the classical technique on its own.

'In the treatment of schizoid patients,' he writes, *(The Maturational Process and the facilitating Environment,* 241) 'the analyst needs to know all about the interpretations that might be made, but he must be able to refrain from being sidetracked into doing this work . . . because the main need is for an unclever ego-support, or a holding. This 'holding', like the task of the mother in infant care acknowledges tacitly the tendency of the patient to disintegrate, to cease to exist, to fall for ever.'

Michael Balint, a Hungarian and a pupil of Ferenczi, refers to patients whose development has been flawed by a basic fault (Balint, 1968) and need, as a result, to be provided with something more powerful than mere words. More recent writers have acknowledged that it is not only the schizoid or borderline or regressed patients who need warmth and holding – perhaps everyone who comes into therapy needs to be held as well as understood.

While the therapist can in no way hope to reproduce the role of the parents in the patient's infancy, she can provide a service which has many similarities to parenting. Lomas (1987) points out that parent and therapist both share 'the sense of commitment, the pride of achievement, the shame of failure, the dilemma about the amount of influence that is justified, the tantalisation of the sexual taboo, the pain of eventual loss of intimacy – all these feelings and many more are the lot of both therapist and parent and are complemented by those of the patient and the child . . . The therapist, like the parent, is at least as important for what she is, as for what she does.' (Lomas, p 71)

It is rare for anyone to find in adult life a person who will take on anything like this kind of responsibility. Friends may listen and be sympathetic but are apt to be distracted by their own problems which, as soon as they think you are done, they may be waiting to tell you all about. Anthony Storr in his short (1989) book on Freud says: 'Most patients seeking psychoanalysis have never experienced from anyone else the kind of long term concern which is offered in psychoanalysis. There is no other situation in life in which one can count on a devoted listener for so many hours. What many patients experience is an awakening of emotions they have never had, rather than a repetition of fantasies from the past.'

So far I have only mentioned psychotherapists who are practising as psychoanalysts, or have remained close to the analytic tradition. But there are other therapists further out on the liberal or interpersonal (soft) wing, who happily dispense altogether with interpretation and the reconstruction of childhood. Perhaps the best known of them is Carl Rogers, whose method is called Client-Centred Therapy. In Rogers' view everything depends on the client-therapist relationship in the here and now. The therapist must present himself as someone who is trustworthy, dependable and genuine in that he is not concealing anything about himself or pretending to be anything that he is not. He should have positive attitudes to his client such as warmth, caring, interest; he should not be distant or aloof. Thirdly he should be able to feel empathy with the client.

Empathy is a word which does not appear in the classical psychoanalytic literature. What does it mean? Rogers defines it as the ability 'to enter fully into the world of his (the client's) feelings and personal meanings. 'Can I,' he asks, 'step into his private world so completely that I lose all desire to evaluate and judge it? Can I enter it so sensitively that I can move about in it freely without trampling on meanings which are precious to him?' And he goes on to quote a client who said to him,

'What I've looked for so hard is for someone to understand.' (Rogers, *On Becoming a Person,* p 53).

This need to feel understood is deeply important for everyone but particularly for the kind of person who seeks psychotherapy. Not feeling understood can make you doubt your sanity, your value as a human being or even your existence. Yet the need to be able to tune in with empathy to another person's feelings seems to have received little attention from analysts. When they do feel the strength of the patient's emotions they tend to call it 'counter-transference' and their instinct is to interpret it, rather than simply to share it.

It will be clear by now that my sympathies lie much more with the soft liberals who see themselves as parent-like figures nurturing their patients, than with the hard line conservatives who are mainly there to interpret. I find the writings of the soft analysts very persuasive and my own patients seem to have changed and improved in response to my 'holding' or 'mothering', rather than to my explanations. But I could be wrong. It may be that application of the classical psychoanalytic technique is actually more effective in increasing self-knowledge and hence self-realisation, as Freud originally maintained. How can we tell?

The hard line conservative analyst might say that the patient's recollections of therapy are irrelevant. 'Aaron Green', the analyst interviewed by Janet Malcolm in *Psychoanalysis: the Impossible Profession,* follows up Freud's surgical analogy by comparing the analytic ex-patient to someone who has had an operation under general anaesthetic. He has no memory of the procedure, but he wakes up cured. In a more poetic mood, 'Aaron' compares the patient to the human characters in *A Midsummer Night's Dream,* who, at the end 'wake up and rub their eyes and are not sure what has happened to them. They have the feeling that a great deal has occurred – and things have somehow changed for the better, but they do not know what caused the change.'

Unfortunately it is very difficult, perhaps impossible, to find an objective way of discovering whether a patient has really changed for the better as a result of psychotherapy. She may appear to be functioning well, to have a good job and a satisfactory relationship, but how do we know that this is due to the treatment and not to the passage of time or the intervention of other factors outside the therapy? It might be more convincing if everyone, or nearly everyone, who has been through psychotherapy was clearly seen to be very much better with no recurrence of their previous trouble. After all, the majority of patients who go through appendicectomy emerge with only a neat scar and have no further problems with that part of their intestine.

Psychotherapy patients, on the other hand, will only too often experience further emotional crises and continue to live lives beset with personal difficulties; they may even need further periods of treatment. Freud himself, in later life, was troubled about the temporary nature of many analytic 'cures' and voiced his doubts in a paper called *Analysis Terminable and Interminable* (Freud, 1937). Perhaps without psychotherapy such people's lives would have been even more difficult (patients will often tell you so) but there is no objective way of measuring that.

The fact is that evaluation of this kind of treatment is a near impossible task – some writers have dismissed it as unworthy of the interest of scientists for this very reason. There is, unfortunately, no good evidence that any kind

126

of dynamic psychotherapy or psychoanalysis is better than any other kind. In these circumstances I think that we ought to listen to what the patients themselves have to say. Clearly their testimony will be subject to all sorts of biases and misconceptions, but in the absence of any objective evidence what thay have to say has to be at least of interest.

Rosemary Dinnage in her book *One to One* (Dinnage, 1988) printed personal accounts by twenty patients or ex-patients, and in her introductory chapter tried to summarise some of the factors which, according to their experience, made for success or failure in therapy.

' "He (or she) liked me!" was the astonished discovery of several patients who linked it with the beginning of liking themselves.' Some talked of 'acquiring a sort of internal helper who stays around for life.' Others attributed improvement to the therapist's personality:

'Strong, healthy, rocklike'; 'real enough to make me feel it is worth being real'; 'he never hid or pretended to be what he was not.' Others, describing what went wrong with their therapy said things like:

'He did not feel safe'; 'she was afraid of me.' One patient, (Philip), says of his Freudian analyst,

'He was a horrible type, . . . sadistic, mocking,' Another patient (Elizabeth) complains that 'there was no friendliness at any point.

'I think ordinary, normal friendliness is part of making you feel like a person rather than something to be processed, a robot. I think I felt I was someone to be beaten through all that time, to have a lot knocked out of me. I feel that most of the time I was surrounded by a torrent of negative interpretations – sometimes in my ignorance I thought I was doing well, but everything was turned on its head. In all the eleven years I cannot remember anything good being said about me . . .'

Of course, it is always possible that an unpleasant experience may ultimately produce a cure: a surgical operation is no picnic even with the benefit of an anaesthetic, and every one knows that the most effective medicine may have a nasty taste. As I have said, objective evaluation of psychotherapy is practically impossible. In the end every therapist has to find his or her own position somewhere between the extremes of hard and soft, and practice in the style that seems to be right for her.

Those who believe strongly in a theory will see the patient's acceptance of those beliefs and ability to use it as an explanation of themselves as the best evidence of clinical improvement. Indeed a patient may often feel much more secure if she is able to see herself in terms of a theological system instead of floundering around unable to 'understand' herself. This benefit may come regardless of whether the theory is true or false or only partly true.

The transformation of the patient's view of herself and her world is akin to a religious conversion – and there is nothing wrong with that. Many people derive great comfort and support from religious beliefs and are able to help others as a result. There are different religions as there are different theories of the mind; they all share some assumptions, while differing in detail. What does it matter? Perhaps the only important thing is that the conversion should not be swiftly followed by disillusionment and a feeling of having been cheated or 'conned', as happens all too often to the followers of extreme religious (and psychotherapeutic) cults. Meanwhile those, like myself, whose tendency is to be agnostic, will feel more comfortable with a more agnostic therapeutic style, less dependent on doctrine than simple human values.

However, even an agnostic is heavily influenced by the

theology of the culture in which he has grown up. I have been steeped in the literature of psychoanalysis for a long time and had nearly five years of psychoanalysis myself. I still find the ideas of Freud and Melanie Klein very appealing, although there is a good deal of detail in their theories that I can no longer take seriously. We owe to psychoanalysis the model of the therapist and patient as a kind of mother (or parent) and child. I find this metaphor for the therapeutic relationship and the business of therapy consistently useful and repeatedly illuminating. Sometimes I share the metaphor with my patient in the form of an interpretation, sometimes I keep it to myself. But I would not like to be without it.

Another concept which comes from psychoanalysis is the idea that when a patient in therapy talks about a third person or an animal or even a force of nature, she may also be talking about a part of herself. The third person might be a friend who makes people feel envious; the animal might be a lost kitten with whose plight the patient identifies; the force of nature might be a storm which echoes and reflects her own turbulent feelings. I am not sure whether psychoanalysis has a technical term which embraces all these phenomena; for me they represent the kind of 'interpretation' which makes immediate sense and facilitates understanding.

I am also prepared to use transference interpretations of a modest kind. I am sure that it is vital not to underestimate one's importance in the patient's mind and heart – I have made this mistake more than once as you will see from the case histories. So if the patient is talking about a close relationship which she is afraid of losing, it may be helpful to ask tentatively if she has the same feelings about her therapist. But this is a long way from assuming that every relationship mentioned by the patient is a disguised reference to the solipsistic therapist.

As for the transference itself, I go along with Anthony Storr (Storr 1989, p 40) when he says that the patient's attitudes to the therapist 'have their history which needs to be explored. But the emphasis is on understanding in what way the patient's attitude to others is distorted through perceiving in what way his attitude to the analyst is distorted. To do this effectively requires that the psychoanalyst is not concerned solely with the events of early childhood, but also recognises that there is a real relationship in the here and now.'

I find that attempts to deny any value or reality to the intrinsic here and now relationship is to deprive the patient of the real presence of the kind-of-parent whom he desperately needs. As Ferenczi says, we must 'take his infantile need for help seriously (and we cannot offer a helpless child, which is what most patients are, mere theories, when it is in terrible pain) . . .' *(Clinical Diaries* p 210). I go along with him and I go along with Winnicott in his wish to 'Hold the patient.'

I suspect with Lomas that Winnicott believed this too, but was too respectful of his psychoanalytical forbears to come out with it. I applaud and feel supported by Winnicott when he says (Winnicott p 167) 'One interpretation per session satisfies me . . . I never use long sentences unless I am very tired. If I am near exhaustion point I begin teaching.'

Finally, in acknowledging the source of my style, I must mention my debt to Carl Rogers for the notion that simply sharing feelings and trying to understand how the other person feels, may be worth any number of intellectually brilliant interpretations.

To summarise: In my role as a part-time psycho-therapist I try to do the following:

1) Offer a small part of my time at regular

intervals for as long as it is needed.

2) Behave responsibly, thoughtfully and, as far as possible, warmly, as if I were a kind of parent or guardian who sees his child only intermittently, but holds her in his mind from each session to the next.

3) Try to share feelings, including the burden of painful ones without complaining or disintegrating.

4) Accept anger without retaliating (but not permit physical violence).

5) Accept love without devaluing it; decline sexual invitations gently but firmly.

6) Make the occasional interpretation when I think the patient is unconsciously using a metaphor.

7) Refer, from time to time, to my role as a kind of parent: and to the emergence in this context of the patient's childhood feelings.

I called this chapter 'How does psychotherapy work?' as if I hoped to provide an answer to the question. The fact is that I do not really know how it works, or even whether it works. But I feel the need to do it all the same. To quote Anthony Storr again, 'Even if it could be proven that psychotherapy was not effective . . . we should still, as physicians, and still more as human beings, be called upon to make some attempt to care for people in distress of mind: and this would inevitably result in our trying to make some relationship with such people. We should therefore be driven into psychotherapy even if we disbelieved in its efficacy: for as I see it psychotherapy consists fundamentally in two people attempting to make a relationship with each other.' (Storr, 1960, *The Integrity of the Personality,* p 128).

131

11

CAN GPS DO PSYCHOTHERAPY?

In my introductory chapter ('Beginnings') I explained how I came to involve myself in formal psychotherapy with patients after surgery hours. I would now like to look at the question of whether it is appropriate for a GP to be doing this kind of work, when there are other professionals who are better trained to do it. Most people nowadays expect their family doctor to be sensitive to their emotional state and able at least to make a start in helping with emotional problems. Having made a disgnosis, we are then expected to refer the patient to someone else, a psychiatrist or a social worker or perhaps a practice counsellor, if one is available. If I mention my interest in psychotherapy to a counsellor or a social worker, I am usually told, 'Of course you do not really have the time for that sort of thing, do you? Your consultations can only last ten minutes at the most and you are always under tremendous pressure.' It is true that we are under pressure in NHS general practice to fit in a lot of people, but this is not entirely a bad thing if it means that we are always accessible and do not make people wait a long time for an appointment. But there is no law that restricts a consultation to a ten minute maximum: most doctors faced with a patient in distress will let the interview run on until she has unburdened herself sufficiently, at least for the time being. Hopefully, the next patient will have only a simple request, such as a repeat prescription or a certificate, and the doctor will be able to catch up a little. We can cope with a certain number of extended consultations, particularly if we feel that we have done a good job and been available when we were needed. Many patients get valuable short term help from their family doctors in this way; and for some, a single encounter with a doctor who is able to tune in to the patient's mood may be strikingly effective. For others a short series of consultations may be needed when affairs are in crisis – after which doctor and patient may hardly see each other for a year or more.

Michael and Enid Balint were the pioneers in facilitating this kind og GP psychotherapy and the Balint groups which they started in the 1950s have been an invaluable training ground for GPs wishing to deepen their understanding of the doctor-patient relationship. In the Balints' earlier writings *(The Doctor, his Patient and the Illness, Psychotherapeutic Techniques in Medicine)* it is evident that at least some of the group members (sometimes described as 'psychotherapeutically-minded') were quite eager to take on patients for more extended periods of treatment, and this was quite acceptable to the group leaders. Later on the Balints and their GP colleagues modified the aims of their training so that the emphasis was on ordinary consultations of a normal length, rather than on hour-long interviews with specially selected patients. They became much more concerned with what can be done in a short time in a consultation where intensity is more important than duraction: hence the title of their next book, *Six Minutes for the Patient.* The long interview, formerly a feature of every case presented, is now described by Michael Balint as 'a foreign body' in

133

general practice, and seems no longer to be regarded as appropriate even for a 'psychotherapeutically-minded' GP.

There is a lot to be said for this refocusing of the GP's attention on to his ordinary consultations; much help can be given to a large number of patients if we can observe and notice our patients' emotions and the effects they have on our own feelings as they talk about their symptoms. It does not require a great deal of extra time in the surgery and a Balint group is the ideal place for learning to improve one's insights and skills.

Nevertheless, there remains on every GP's list, a substantial number of patients for whom this is not going to be enough. Who, if not the GP, is going to be the person to help them? Should they be referred as soon as possible to someone with more time and more training? A doctor who is not very interested in patients' personal problems might arrange a referral (eg. to a psychiatrist or social worker) at the first hint of anything to do with upset feelings. But most of us, I think, would ask the patient to come back two or three times to get a better idea of the problem, if only to write a better referral letter. By this time, if doctor and patient have discovered some affinity for each other, it may be getting a little difficult to send the patient to a specialist. The doctor will want to stay in touch and the patient will feel rejected if she is 'passed on' to someone else. She may, after all, have decided to confide in her GP precisely because she recognises her as someone she feels she can trust. This is the point where the interested and sympathetic GP will feel the urge to offer herself as the patient's psychotherapist – and also the point where a number of problems and dangers begin to loom up.

To start with, there are the practical problems. Patients having psychotherapy need to feel that they can rely on a high degree of privacy if they are going to share their feelings and perhaps their tears. If the consulting room is poorly sound-proofed, or the session interrupted by the telephone, or the doctor's secretary keeps running in with a prescription to be signed – then these conditions are not going to be met. The setting will not be right and both therapist and patient will be ill at ease. Having the psychotherapy session at the end of the surgery (the last appointment) will go a long way towards solving the problem as, by that time, the rest of the day's business can have been completed. Even so, it is advisable to make sure that the practice receptionist (who might also be working late) is aware that these consultations should not be interrupted except in dire emergency. Secondly, the temptation to offer psychotherapy sessions too often or to too many people, must be strongly, if regretfully, resisted. Psychotherapy cannot be allowed to encroach on ordinary practice time – that would be unfair to the other patients and to the doctor's partners who would have to shoulder more than their share of the clinical work load. Doing a psychotherapy session means that I shall be home late and I have to decide how many evenings a week I (and my family) are prepared to let this happen. (The answer is not usually more than twice.) Trying to do too much psychotherapy may lead to emotional and physical exhaustion and deprives the doctor of the restoring effect of being with his family, who, in any case, need him just as much as he needs them. Thirdly, I think it is vitally important to have some advice on how to go about structuring the sessions and some supervision of one's work. Having a brother to talk to on a regular basis about the patients had prevented me from feeling prematurely disheartened by slow progress, or totally overwhelmed by the worry and responsibility. I have also found my personal therapy very helpful but I would not go so far as to say that this was absolutely necessary for every GP psychotherapist.

And so, if the doctor is interested enough to make a commitment and the patient is willing, I think a case can be made for the GP to act as a formal psychotherapist for a few of her own patients within the practice. She will need to provide an appropriate setting and sufficient time, and take care not to let herself take on too many patients at once. She will need support and supervision from an experienced psychotherapist and will be considerably helped by the experience of personal therapy, if she can afford it. She will have to be prepared to go on for a number of years with each patient and will be wise to offer therapy only to those patients she feels she can spend a lot of time with, without becoming bored or irritated. But if these conditions are satisfied, GP psychotherapy has much to recommend it. The patient gets time and attention within the practice without having to undergo lengthy assessments and then wait for a therapist to have a vacancy. At the end of the wait, the psychotherapist provided by the NHS may well be a registrar or social worker in training – with less experience than the GP psychotherapist. And even if a good therapeutic relationship is established it may be abruptly broken off because the therapist is moving to take up another career post. GPs, on the other hand, tend to stay in the same post for many years.

Practice counsellors are an alternative solution and a number of practices have found the presence of an attached counsellor very useful. Unfortunately, counsellors are still very thin on the ground because no satisfactory agreement has yet been reached with the Department of Health about paying them. Most of the existing ones are funded by research grants or work on a voluntary basis, supplemented by small contributions from the patients. Good psychotherapy is, of course, available on a private basis in London and other big cities, but only at a cost that most of our patients could not possibly afford.

Since psychotherapy is such a scarce resource one might think that the professionals would be pleased to see some General Practitioners eager to help their own patients in this way. In fact, a number of psycho-therapists I have talked to were very uneasy about the idea of my giving therapy to my own patients, despite the precautions I have described above. Most of their reservations have to do with the subject of transference. Transference is Freud's term for the feelings and attachments of the patient which properly belong to her childhood relationship with her parents, but becomes transferred to the therapist. Freud at first saw transference as an obstacle to the patient's enlighten-ment, but later realised that it was actually helpful in that the patient's feelings became more directly accessible if they were about the analyst himself. Transference feelings seem to be aroused very readily towards anyone who extends a helping hand or offers a sympathetic ear. They are very powerful and easily underestimated by the novice. Inexperienced doctors of any speciality may fail to recognise how important they have become to their patients even in a very short period of contact. The doctor may fail to anticipate the distress or anger which can be provoked by a holiday or even 'I will see you in a month's time' instead of the expected 'same time next week.' Patients may suffer intense jealousy over a doctor who becomes pregnant or gives any indication of enjoying her family life. Not infrequently, the patient's transference becomes quite erotic, and she may have all sorts of fantasies in which her love for her doctor is reciprocated. These phenomena can cause big problems

137

for the specialist psychotherapist, but at least he can avoid physical contact with his patients. The GP, on the other hand, in the course of his ordinary clinical care of the patient may need to examine her, to see her naked, even to insert instruments into her openings. What wild fantasies might this sort of thing evoke in a patient already regressed and excited by transference feelings? The psychotherapist shudders and declares that the whole thing is impossible, unthinkable. All I can say is that in practice this sort of reaction has never seemed to be a problem. Most of my psychotherapy patients are very healthy physically, and soon lose their psycho-somatic symptoms once they enter into regular therapy. When they do get respiratory infections, I listen to their chests, whether male or female, and nothing very dramatic appears to happen. If a woman patient requires a vaginal examination (for example for a cervical smear test) she will usually, though not invariably, go to one of my female partners. The one patient who did develop an intense sexual desire for me was never examined physically at all.

But even without these physical encounters, the GP, it is argued, is unable to function as a blank screen reflecting her patients' impressions of her while revealing nothing of herself. In her surgery, doing her house calls, perhaps even on show in the supermarket or at the village fete, she is all too obviously a real person whose life can be observed and known about. I can answer this objection only by saying that I have never been troubled by the need to be like a blank screen or even a polished mirror, and I am not aware that my visibility as a real person has ever interfered with the kind of therapy that I practice.

We now come to counter-transference, which always accompanies transference and is inter-twined with it.

The relationship with the patient engenders feelings in the therapist which may have profound effects: diagnostic, therapeutic or disruptive. The GP therapist needs to be aware that some of the feelings he experiences will have been planted in his head by the patient. We have all had encounters with people who have made us feel guilty, or angry or profoundly sad, often without our realising at first, what is going on. More dangerously for the therapist, she may be particularly disturbed or excited by a patient who has problems similar to some of her own unresolved personal difficulties. I have already said that we GP psychotherapists offer therapy to those patients for whom we feel an affinity, and I would maintain that this common ground can be the foundation of an effective therapeutic relationship. It is also possible for us to become closely involved with a patient without recognising that we share his problems, and this can result in an unhealthy collusion in which the therapist is using the patient to satisfy his own needs. I have to ask myself if I would be able to recognise if this was going to happen and whether I would be able to prevent it. There have been occasions, mainly with 'the boys' when I have been tempted to cross too far over the professional boundary and this may have been an indication of unconscious collusion. It does not seem to have happened with any of my fully established psychotherapy patients, although I cannot be certain, and it may be apparent in the case histories: the reader must judge.

Finally, even if she can avoid the pitfalls of transference and counter-transference in the surgery, the GP therapist may still be charged with sheer lack of resources. She may succeed in opening up some sensitive areas, break down the patient's defences and then be unable to contain the patient's helplessness and fear. If a patient is seen only once a week, it may be argued, and she becomes deeply regressed, the GP setting does not provide sufficient strength or containment for her to be held and comforted as she could be in five-times-a-week therapy or in a hospital. A GP is in no position to step up the number of sessions and has no direct access to hospital beds – although hospital colleagues may well be able to help in an emergency. I have described the occasion when this happened in my own practice in the case history of Margaret. This is a serious problem and deserves some consideration; as in any other branch of medicine or professional helping, it is important to be able to call on specialist help and advice when it is required. But the overriding question is whether at the end of the day the psychotherapeutic endeavour is seen to have been helpful, or harmful, or perhaps neither. Evaluation of psychotherapy is notoriously difficult but we can at least establish a few criteria.

How could one tell if psychotherapy was going seriously wrong for a patient? What sort of events or changes in her life would one look for objectively? The most serious would be death by suicide, although even this might not be preventable in a depressed and determined patient. Secondly, the patient's mental structure might begin to collapse with signs of psychotic illness such as delusions, thought disorders and disconnection from external reality. I have described how this happened to one of my patients (Margaret), and I have no doubt that it resulted from my ill-advised decision to lengthen the intervals between her sessions. Nevertheless, it was possible, with a little help from my psychiatric colleagues, to rescue Margaret, and her subsequent progress has been encouraging.

A patient might also make foolish or impulsive decisions under the influence of her therapist, which

140

would be damaging to her life. She might give up a good job or leave a marriage, to the detriment of her children; or become homeless or financially insecure for other reasons. One of my patients (Louise) lost her job during therapy and had difficulty in getting another one at the same level. Other patients either found jobs (of varying degrees of satisfaction) or continued to be unemployed. One patient (Duncan) left his family a few years after therapy finished and this caused me some distress at the thought of his abandoned wife and children. The others either found partners (Margaret, Sally, Louise) or remained single. Finally, one might say that a patient who becomes totally dependent on her GP therapist has been harmed or damaged in that she has been prevented from developing independently. This might be evident if the patient was constantly haunting the surgery seeking appointments and in general spending more time with doctors than she did before the therapy started. One of my patients (Margaret again) has found great difficulty in separating from me and that caused me some anxiety at the time. But subsequent events showed that she and I still had some important work to attend to, and the extended time scale was needed to complete it.

So according to the best criteria I can think of (readers may think of others) I do not see that there is much evidence of harm or damage resulting to the patients from my efforts to help them. A few disappointments, perhaps, but no disasters. And it is worth remembering that the potential disasters I have mentioned can, and do, sometimes happen to specialist psychotherapists.

GP psychotherapy, at least as practised by me, has apparently not done any significant damage to the patients concerned. But that is not much to show for all those hours of work that they and I have put in over seventeen years. How can I tell whether they received any positive benefits from those hours they spent in my consulting room? I will try to address this problem in my final chapter. But, before that, I would like to have a look at the reasons why I found myself working with these particular patients, rather than some of the others who needed help, perhaps just as badly.

12

CHEMISTRY

It is clear that a GP psychotherapist cannot hope to offer this kind of service to more than a small number of patients in a professional lifetime. This raises the question of how the patients are selected. How can the doctor determine which of the many troubled and damaged patients in her practice population are going to be the ones who will repay the investment of many hours of her time, and a good deal of worry and concern? When I started I did not have any criteria for choosing patients. I offered myself as a psychotherapist to people whom I liked, felt sad for, and felt I could get along with without becoming bored. To some extent they probably chose me; they brought their problems to me instead of another partner or another practice. Some of them I ignored at first, but they kept on coming back to me until I took them seriously. Why did they pick me? Perhaps I had certain characteristics of personality which appealed to them and facilitated the emergence of transference feelings. Similarly, I may have found in their personalities something which strongly evoked a counter-transference in me which made me respond to them more positively.

Counter-transference feelings are considered by

psychotherapists to have both virtues and dangers. Their presence can be an aid to diagnosis in that the emotions evoked in the therapist may be a valuable clue to the way the patient is feeling at the moment (Heiman, 1950). On the other hand, it is argued, if the patient's plight awakens feelings in the therapist which really belong to his own unresolved problems, he may be unable to treat the patient with appropriate distance and objectivity.

It becomes apparent that the therapist's response to her patient's personality is a very complex matter. It becomes possible to like a patient on the surface, at the conscious level, but find him profoundly disturbing at a deeper level because he stirs up one's own unconscious conflicts. Conversely, a doctor may find himself strongly drawn to and fascinated by a patient whom he does not at first find very interesting or likeable. With most of our patients in General Practice, there is little opportunity to pick and choose and, fortunately for them, it is quite possible to treat many patients' problems effectively, whether one likes them or not, and without getting too much entangling of their feelings and our own. But when there is something more at stake than an easily disposed of symptom; when emotion begins to be invested in the need for relief and understanding, it is a different matter. Doctors can choose the extent to which they get involved and will often instinctively keep their emotional distance if they perceive, consciously or unconsciously, that letting their feelings be engaged will result in discomfort. At other times, or with other patients, a doctor may decide that he will become more involved. When the doctor is young and inexperienced, allowing his own feelings to be stirred by a patient can be upsetting, both professionally and personally. He may find himself in urgent need of some help if the therapeutic relationship is to prosper, and one of the best ways of getting help is, in my view, to join a Balint group. These case discussion groups for GPs were started by Michael and Enid Balint in London in the 1950s and they have since become internationally recognised and reproduced. I have spent ten years as a Balint group leader in a GP training course and have listened to many young doctors telling the stories of their struggle to understand their patients' emotional turmoil. One thing that has struck me (and many of my colleagues e.g. Samuel, 1988) is the way in which the same doctor will present a series of patients with whom he is having difficulties, all of whom have characteristics in common. The way in which 'Dr A presents the same patient over and over again' is often apparent to the other members of the group long before Dr A himself realises what is going on. Sometimes it is only the group leaders who notice that Dr A is actually presenting himself, or aspects of himself which trouble him, and are reflected in the problems and emotional disturbances of his chosen patients. It would seem that when he looks into the inner world of one of these patients, he sees an image of himself there, staring back. The basis for this identification may be quite obvious: for example when patient and doctor are of a similar age, sex and social background. The doctor may even have had to cope with a very similar crisis, such as a bereavement or a divorce, in the recent past. At other times, the characteristics that doctor and patient have in common may be hidden and unexpected. Then the recognition takes place at an unconscious level; the doctor finds himself preoccupied with the patient without really knowing why.

Sometimes, when I hear a doctor talking about his patient in a Balint group, I get the impression that the two of them have something in common which is rather too painful for the doctor; perhaps a feeling of rejection or humiliation. When this is happening, the doctor hesitates to get more deeply involved. Having recognised something of himself in the patient, he finds the mirror image so repellant that he wants to escape, although he remains curious and fascinated. Instead of helping the patient directly, he may try to refer him to someone else, such as a social worker or counsellor: usually to no avail, because the patient, who also recognises a kindred spirit when he sees one, keeps coming back to the doctor!

On the other hand, the doctor's empathy and sense of identification may be so powerful that he plunges head first into the patient's world and tries to merge with him. Group leaders learn to recognise this sort of problem too, and become alert for the danger signals: the doctor spends an increasing amount of time with the patient; consultations become longer and increase in frequency, sometimes to more than once a day. Home visits are also increased, although the patient may be quite fit enough to come to the surgery. The professional boundary becomes blurred and may vanish altogether as the doctor becomes 'more like a friend.' He fights the patient's battles for him on every front, neglecting himself and his family. He may also fail to realise that the patient is becoming psychotic and really needs admission to hospital.

Somewhere in between these extremes of repulsion and total immersion, lies the ideal professional relationship between a hurt patient and a doctor who can feel similar wounds in his own psyche. The pain is not so bad as to be unbearable, and the patient is not rejected; but the doctor is able to keep his own identity separate and look after his own needs, as well as caring for those of the patient. If these requirements are met, then the therapeutic alliance can prosper.

Patients presented in Balint discussion groups may be

seen only once or twice before contact is lost or broken off. But quite often they are seen regularly over a long period of time and it is apparent that doctor and patient are engaging in a form of psychotherapy. I feel sure that similar processes of recognition and identification must have operated in my own decisions to get involved with certain patients in a psychotherapeutic relationship. I have called this chapter 'Chemistry' because I see the mutual recognition of doctor and patient as a slightly mysterious process, a bit like falling in love, which does not happen in accordance with common sense or prudence, regrettable as this may seem. Chance brought certain patients into my consulting room – and chemistry did the rest. Chemical (emotional) affinity became apparent: they knew I was the one to help them and I knew they were the people I wanted to help.

However, the chemistry needs to be studied. Chemical substances can be slightly unstable and some of their reactions may be explosive. What exactly are these qualities that my patients and I have in common? How many of them are desirable? Are they qualities we can be proud of or do we share some secrets that we would both prefer to keep hidden? It is well known that doctors and patients can collude with each other in suppressing painful subjects such as addiction to alcohol, or the nearness of death, and while this may lead to cosy intimacy it is not going to be therapeutic in the long run. I hope that such collusions and evasions have not undermined my psychotherapeutic work, but I cannot be sure.

Now let me turn to the patients described in the case histories and look for ways in which we mirror and match each other, in order to illustrate the part counter-transference can play in the client (patient) – counsellor (doctor) relationship.

147

DUNCAN had a bright intellect, enjoyed literature and wanted to improve himself academically, all of which evoked positive responses in me. My wish to help is very easily enlisted by anyone wanting to take an examination or apply for a place in college. In arguments I often express contempt for academic qualifications and academic 'excellence'; but I spent the best years of my youth in pursuit of them so perhaps (secretly) I value them highly. As a person, Duncan was solitary, withdrawn and gloomy: not a condition I enjoy very much. But he did have a sharply ironic sense of humour which provided us with a good deal of shared pleasure. And he also shared my covert yearning to be spoiled and petted a little (without of course admitting it). He often felt that his life was fairly pointless and might as well be ended. I did not really share that feeling, but I do sometimes enter a state of mind in which although life is tolerable, even enjoyable at times, it would not really matter if it was extinguished. So I did not find his nihilistic ruminations alien or intolerable.

SALLY was quite different. She made persistent, impudent demands for my attention and recognition of her sexuality, in a way that I would never have done. Perhaps her shameless attention-seeking appealed to me because I could experience it vicariously. And to be the object of such urgent needs was obviously flattering. She also tested my ability to keep both of us under control, although I think her ability to see the funny side of her desire and my anxiety also made me warm to her.

MARGARET was the only one who was in no sense an intellectual. Her job was a fairly mechanical one and she had no desire to take examinations, go on courses or acquire qualifications. She was sad and lonely (like

Duncan but without his arrogance and wit.) She was clinging and adhesive, determined, like Sally, to get my attention, but without Sally's cheekiness. Certainly she was another outsider longing to find someone with whom she could share affection. She achieved more than I expected because she hung on and would not let me go: on the other hand I could have shaken her off if I had been more ruthless. Perhaps I need constantly to be reminded of the anxious and reproachful feelings of people who depend on me, if I am not to turn my back on them.

The other three patients were more ambivalent about their need for me. HELEN seemed to come reluctantly to her sessions like a sulky child to a boring lesson. At the same time she had two powerful counter-transference effects on me. One was to make me feel protective and fearful about her potential for committing suicide. I suppose any doctor would be worried about a young girl killing herself before she had really had a chance to live, so probably this was not something which had to fit exactly with anything special in me. The second effect was to make me feel excluded from a relationship she was having with someone else: the odd one out in a triangle. I think this was something that she herself experienced and wanted unconsciously to project into me, as the Kleinian terminology has it. If this was so, it found a secure place to lodge; I could easily accept that excluded feeling as something that belonged to me. On the other hand, it was not so uncomfortable that I had to reject it and her. Instead, I allowed her to treat me with aloofness and disdain for much of the time – and felt quite a keen pleasure on those occasions when she allowed me to share her more private feelings, or was just a little bit concerned about me.

I shall move on to JENNIFER. She appealed to me first because of her bright and brittle gaiety, her confident sparkle with which was blended vulnerability and pathos. Like me, she was afraid of the gulf that might open up if she allowed herself to become too dependent on someone. We had this in common, but in the end it made her run away from me after a relatively short time in therapy.

Finally, there was LOUISE, who like most of the others was very intelligent and highly educated. She had an appearance of cheerful, aggressive confidence which I found exhilarating. But when we talked, the facade would easily crumble, revealing a tearful little girl who had never understood what happened when her father died. I never suffered that kind of loss, but I can show a confident face to the world, feel successful, secure and wanted. And yet, I only have to suffer a reverse of some sort in my professional life to feel small, lost and insignificant. I do not think I fly from this feeling in such a panic as Louise did, so I felt I could hold some of it for her. I was happy to stay with her, but she found the dependent feelings painful, and she decided not to come back!

CONCLUSION

My little group of patients were by no means photocopies of each other or of me. But I think I can find enough features familiar from my own internal world to convince me that we did have important things in common. The point I would like to make in conclusion is that the phenomenon of doctors choosing patients with whom they have a 'chemical' affinity to work with is so common that it may even be an essential element in psychotherapy. In other words, psychotherapy may not work without the chemistry. I would disagree with those who say that a therapist cannot work effectively with patients who affect him in this way, while I recognise that problems, even disasters, can occur if the therapist is insufficiently aware of what is going on. If he does have sufficient awareness he will be able to prevent himself from becoming over-involved. If the involvement is just right and the therapeutic distance appropriate, there is the prospect of a real working relationship between two people whose 'chemistry' is right for each other.

13

EVALUATION AND FOLLOW UP

In this final chapter, I would like to examine some of the positive gains that one might hope for as a result of this sort of psychotherapy and see how far those hopes have been fulfilled by the patients I have described.

People are offered psychotherapy as a way of relieving psychic pain. As well as being unpleasant to experience, this kind of pain interferes with the rest of one's life. Work becomes arduous or impossible, and personal relationships disintegrate. Unable to comfort himself, the person in psychic pain is unlikely to be able to help anyone else, and this lack of usefulness may be a further source of pain.

Psychic pain seems to have two main components, at least as doctors perceive and describe it today. These are the well-known symptoms of anxiety and depression. The writers of helpful psychiatric articles for GPs emphasise the importance of recognising and differentiating these states, and the pharmaceutical companies provide a copious supply of drugs for the relief of both.

Unfortunately, anxiety and depression have a way of persisting even when they have been recognised and prescribed for, as my psychotherapy patients discovered.

Depression embraces a wide variety of feelings including persisting sadness or misery, feelings of guilt or worthlessness, and a sense of inner emptiness or barrenness of the spirit. Anxiety is a more restless kind of unhappiness: its manifestations include panic attacks, nameless dreads, constant worries and doubts about problems from the trivial to the cosmic; fears of being alone or overwhelmed by crowds; and physical symptoms such as sweating, trembling and palpitation.

Can psychotherapy really relieve this kind of distress? And how can we demonstrate that this has happened? The most obvious way is to ask the patient, do you feel better? And do you think the improvement is due to your treatment with the psychotherapist? The second question is necessary because people may also feel better spontaneously or as a result of other events or encounters which have nothing to do with the therapy. Both questions are flawed, as instruments of evaluation by the possibility of bias in the patient's reply; he may want to give the impression that he feels better as a result of his therapy in order not to disappoint the therapist who has worked so hard for him. In addition we must remember that no-one who has spent several years and perhaps a lot of money on psychotherapy will want to admit, even to himself, that it was all wasted.

A more objective way to assess subjective improval is to ask the patient to complete a standard questionnaire which has been validated by testing it on groups of 'normal' people and other groups, (usually hospital patients), who are known to be depressed or anxious. These questionnaires incorporate numerical scales so that the degree of severity of the symptoms may be quantified. If the psychotherapy patients are tested before and after treatment one might be able to say whether any statistically significant change in their scores had occurred. Similarly one could record patients' consumption of medication or the frequency of their ordinary visits to the GP before and after treatment, to see if there has been any change for the better. All these methods yield results which can be expressed numerically which always makes a better impression on the scientific community that anecdotal reports.

But they too have their problems of interpretation. Many people are found to be at their worst if their mood is sampled immediately before they come for help. They are caught in the middle of a crisis which might be going to settle one way or another whether they have therapy or not. A year later they might be feeling better and produce better test scores with or without the benefit of therapy. The answer to this problem is to perform a controlled trial in which two groups of closely matched patients are compared: one group receives the psychotherapy being tested, while the other receives no treatment or perhaps a placebo therapy. Trials of this kind have been very useful in testing the effectiveness of new antibiotics or drugs for the control of high blood pressure. But human misery is not as standardised as bronchitis or blood pressure: individual differences are considerable. The treatment takes a long time and large numbers are needed to demonstrate any statistically significant difference. So far, despite a lot of hard work and ingenuity, there are no convincing proofs, using these impeccably scientific methods, that psychotherapy does or does not work.

Despite the difficulty, or perhaps impossibility, of obtaining a scientific evaluation of my six patients, I wanted to see what had happened to them a few years down the road, and to make some attempt to assess the work we had done together. After all, a lot of time and effort had gone into it on their part as well as mine. If it had all been wasted or misdirected, I thought, it would be preferable for me to face this disagreeable conclusion and try to learn from my mistakes.

I thought about standardised tests for depression and so forth, but soon decided against them, mainly because I had no pre-therapy scores with which to compare them. Instead I decided to send each patient a questionnaire of my own devising to get an idea of their own subjective evaluation of the therapy, and to supplement this with an assessment of their wellbeing on the basis of a number of purely factual criteria of social functioning. Always assuming that the state of their inner world would have some influence on their ability to lead lives that were creative, useful and enjoyable, at least some of the time. After much thought I decided on a list of six areas of functioning which seemed to me both important and measurable. I will list them and then discuss each in turn.

THE SIX CRITERIA
Work
Love
Other relationships
Learning
Helping others
Independence

1) WORK. Freud declared that the most important things in life were 'Love and Work,' and I am happy to include both in my list. Most people seem to have a need to work which is only partly to do with getting paid. Even without the need to earn a living, a perpetual holiday would make most of us restless; we want to be involved in some way with something, doing something, helping someone; meshing with the purposeful activity of the rest of the

community. It is hard to do this if you are anxious or depressed or afraid of meeting people. So I think it is reasonable to regard starting a job and sticking to it, or progressing to a more challenging kind of work as a sign of improved emotional health.

2) LOVE. Several of my patients complained of feeling unloved, having no-one to love and no partner with whom to share their lives. Sometimes they made me feel like a hard-pressed marriage broker with the urgency of their need, and they left me in no doubt that love and perhaps marriage would be their idea of a successful outcome to their therapy. But love affairs can be transient and marriages disastrous; it would seem unwise to count either in themselves as signs of health or happiness. However, if a previously lonely patient is seen to have developed a loving relationship which seems to be lasting and harmonious, I would feel justified in awarding her (and her therapist) a lot of points.

3) OTHER RELATIONSHIPS. No other relationship can compare with being in love, especially if it lasts; but for some of us, unhappily, it just does not happen, or it does not last. Less intense relationships with other people can still be enjoyable and satisfying – if you are able to connect with them. My patients often complained about having no-one to talk to, and no friends; or only the kind of friends who make enemies superfluous. Some were too shy or lacking in self-confidence to reach out to other people; others too easily alienated potential friends by their moody or suspicious behaviour. Some people are very self-contained and are happy with their own company for long periods: on the whole they do not seem to seek psychotherapy. But most of us feel happier if we have someone to talk to and can relate without too much tension to the people we meet socially and at work.

4) LEARNING. Improving one's education is closely related to work, but I have listed it separately because a number of my patients seemed to think it was especially important. They were eager to develop themselves intellectually or make up for past failures, or just move into the kind of environment where learning was more highly valued. In order to learn you have to be curious and interested in what other people have said and written; this is difficult if you are in constant pain, preoccupied with inner problems or unwilling to accept any kind of outside help.

To move up the educational ladder it is necessary to take and pass examinations; this requires a degree of commitment and self-discipline which is impossible for those in mental anguish. On the other hand it is possible to be good at passing examinations and intellectually successful while neglecting one's inner life and sealing off one's emotional communication channels with other people. I do not like the idea of psychotherapy as a process for helping people to gain academic success at the cost of emotional starvation (although this may have happened to some extent). But it is probably impossible to succeed academically if you are a total mess emotionally. Educational progress is one of my criteria then, but in the absence of other signs of improvement, one to be treated with caution.

5) HELPING OTHERS. Psychological ill-health, or just plain unhappiness, tends to make people preoccupied with themselves and without much energy or motivation left for alleviating the distress of others. Occasionally, I am a little alarmed when someone I regard as quite sick, announces that she is going to train as some kind of fringe therapist. People may attempt to deal with their own problems by 'helping' other people with similar problems. I think this need has a lot to do with attracting

157

quite competent people (like me) into the helping professions, but hopefully we are not too sick to distinguish between our patients' needs and our own. If I think one of my patient's desire to help is premature or misdirected, I try tactfully to point this out. But if, after a period of therapy, I can see a sustained and responsible involvement in helping other people in any way, either practically or by listening to their problems, I regard it as a sign of growth.

6) INDEPENDENCE. I have in mind the ability to be free of undue dependence on either substances or other people. The word 'substance' is now used to include medical drugs of addictive potential, such as heroin; alcohol or other social drugs such as cannabis or tobacco; and other chemicals such as glue or solvents, which may be used as a form of instant (though short-lived) oblivion, by people in distress. Some substances (like tobacco) are more harmful than others; some are harmless when used carefully (alcohol) but disastrous when they take over someone's life. All of them tend to offer a sort of readily accessible comfort and denial of responsibility, which obviates the need to put one's trust in fragile links with other human beings. The addict feels insecure in his inner world and distrustful of help from others – especially if it involves giving up his precious 'substance.' So I think it is reasonable to see the ability to do without these chemical comforters, or at least to use them sparingly, as a sign of progress towards health.

But what about excessive dependence on another person? Healthy adult life depends on the ability to function without parents and, according to analytic theory, this is achieved by internalising the helpful and protective functions of the parents as experienced in childhood. Psychotherapy provides a supplementary dose of parenting, but what happens if this is never successfully absorbed? What if the patient is happy and able to function socially but only with the help of a permanent therapist 'parent'? If the patient's life continues to be centred on her therapist after a reasonable period of treatment (I do not know how long that is, but I should have thought that five years was enough for most people), then one might argue that the appearance of independence was illusory.

We must also remember that some people are unable to develop sufficient dependence on the therapist in the first place to allow much to be achieved. Others break off prematurely, fearful of getting out of their depth in such warm water. Remaining untouched by the experience of therapy is hardly a mark of success. So progress according to this criterion requires evidence of a healthy trust in the therapist followed by a successful emancipation: much as successful child rearing involves close nurturing followed by weaning and gradual progress to adult independence.

THE QUESTIONNAIRE

In designing the questionnaire I tried to give the patients an opportunity to describe the present state of their lives and feelings and to relate any change to the therapy, if they felt this was appropriate. I also wanted to give them a chance to express any negative or regretful feelings about the time they spent with me (while being aware that they might wish to spare my feelings.) The questions were as follows:

> 1) How do you feel about yourself and the way your life is going at the present time? How does this compare with the way you were in the year

159

before the therapy started?

2) Was the experience of therapy helpful? If so, in what way? Has it influenced the direction of your life?

3) Do you think the therapy was bad for you in any way?

4) Have you any regrets about the therapy?

5) Is there anything else you would like to say about it?

PERSONAL FOLLOW UP

The third element in my assessment package was an unstructured talk with the patients about how they were getting on and what they were doing. This was not possible in every case, but was particularly valuable for those with whom I had not maintained contact since the formal therapy ended.

RESULTS: WHAT HAPPENED TO THE PATIENTS?

DUNCAN. I had heard nothing from Duncan for about eight years. In order to try and track him down, I wrote to his university, asking for my letter to be passed on to the head of his old department, who I thought might be able to tell me about his career as an undergraduate, even if he had lost touch with him since then. To my great delight, I received a reply from one of the lecturers who was able to tell me that Duncan had finished his degree course and achieved a very good upper second class degree, on the strength of which he was awarded a two year scholarship to do research for an M.A. Unfortunately he did not complete this work, (I wonder what happened), and after acquiring a postgraduate teaching qualification he found a job teaching languages in a comprehensive school. The lecturer adds: 'He and I became good friends and still meet from time to time when he comes to visit. Any personal details would be better coming from him, so if you wish to contact him, his address is . . . .'

Naturally I wrote to him at once asking for news. In his reply Duncan told me that he was enjoying teaching 'some of the time'. He said he felt that schools and colleges probably did more harm than good, but his colleagues were surprisingly pleasant, and when he had a good lesson (about once a fortnight) he felt 'high enough to get me through all the bad and indifferent ones in between.' His letter continued: 'but what I live for, apart from personal relationships, is playing the piano. It is the one thing that I have ever persevered at and worked really hard at – still not very good, but getting better and I love playing.' He visits his children once a fortnight and the eldest is about to go to university. 'I see Molly from time to time and she seems to be well. That seems to be about it. Strange how few words are needed to summarise eight or nine years. I had thought there would be more to say. I visit the children, play the piano, read, teach and go to the pubs in the evening. Not too bad, really.'

SALLY. Unfortunately, I have no long term follow up and no feedback from Sally herself. I have heard nothing from her or about her since she left the district ten years ago and can only apply my criteria to the way she was then.

At that time, certainly, everything seemed to be going well for her. She was about to take up a new job in her chosen profession. She was in love, engaged and about to be married. She was not taking any drugs and had weaned herself very successfully from a strongly erotic attachment to me. I do not know whether she was able to use her gains in personal strength to help other people. It is impossible to say whether she continued to pursue the positive and hopeful course on which she was set ten years ago or whether any of her partially resolved personal problems caused her further difficulties. Perhaps they did, but if so, I think there is fairly good reason to believe that she had the resources to seek appropriate help and build on the work that she did with me. Meanwhile I am pursuing one or two leads and still hope to get in touch with her again one day.

HELEN. No news from Helen either. This is not really surprising as she showed quite clearly that she wanted to keep me at a distance. The last entry in her medical notes, (for a minor illness), was made by my partner two years ago. At one stage, I heard that she was living in a village in the Cotswolds during the week and returning to stay with her mother at weekends. I wrote to her mother, asking for news; there was no reply and I subsequently discovered that she too had moved away. I telephoned Directory Enquiries who were able to tell me that Helen's name was listed in the area where I had heard she was living: but the telephone number was ex-directory. So the trail has gone cold; and I do not think Helen would really welcome any further attempts to find her. I am left to be comforted only by the thought, already expressed at the end of Helen's chapter, that I may have kept her alive or emotionally viable during a year of crisis. I will not attempt any kind of further evaluation.

MARGARET. Twelve months after the end of the case history our long sessions continue at six week intervals. She has stuck to her job throughout the time I have known her and her employers seem very satisfied with her. After years of loneliness, she found a love partner and, despite the problems described in the case history, they are still together. Recently she has talked about wanting to have a baby and her hopes that it is not too late.

As a result of her relationship with Richard, she has met a number of other people, including his sister and brother-in-law, who seem to have accepted her very easily as a friend. She has a difficult relationship with Richard's mother, but this is hardly surprising. I think that she still finds it hard to exchange small talk with people at work, and tends to be shy and embarrassed with people she does not know. Her dependence on drugs has gradually diminished as a result of her own wish to be free of them. She has stopped her anti-depressants and now takes only a small does of valium at night. She does not smoke and no longer drinks excessively. She is still quite dependent on me in the sense that any suggestion of stopping the sessions completely would be profoundly disturbing. But there is reason to think that we can continue increasing the interval between sessions until eventually they stop. Even if they never stop, her 'dependence' does not incon-venience me or encroach very much on my availability to other patients. It seems a small price to pay for the gains she has made in becoming independent in other ways.

In her reply to the questionnaire Margaret wrote:

> 'I feel happy about the way my life is going at present; much more fulfilling than it used to be. I get less depressed than I used to. The year before therapy I was finding it very difficult to cope with life, feeling suicidal at times, depressed most of the time. The experience of therapy was very helpful in that it helped me to trust someone again. I found that it helped me to understand myself better and to be understood. Therapy changed the direction of my life completely from a gay life to a heterosexual life and I am 100 per cent sure of my sexuality now. I would not say therapy is bad in any way but I found it very painful at times and also found it difficult to be weaned off the therapy as I found the dependency difficult. I am grateful that I was given the chance to have therapy and the time to sort myself out.'

LOUISE. Poor Louise is still struggling. I saw her a few months after our last long session for a minor physical illness, and found that she was still short of money, working hard at a tedious job and unable to find one appropriate for her energy and talents. She had not really begun to 'work' on mourning her mother and this I thought was in some way preventing her from making any progress in getting a 'proper' job in the external world. As usual, I offered her some more sessions but she declined.

I asked her to fill in the questionnaire but she said she

'could not possibly cope with it at the moment.' I sent her another one through the post but received no reply. Judging by my criteria, Louise's outcome looked disappointing. She had made no progress with work, either internal or external. She said nothing encouraging about her social relationships: her friends seemed to have deserted her or been deserted themselves. She was still with her boyfriend and he may turn out to be her life partner, although this was never part of the plan in the days when she really felt in control of her destiny. She is not really in a position to help anyone else and she has made no educational progress. She still smokes heavily but is not dependent on other substances and certainly keeps away from me, except when simple GP services are now and then needed. However, my gloomy feelings about Louise were somewhat lightened when she turned up at the surgery not long ago. I asked how she was and she said: 'Terrible' – but she actually looked quite cheerful.

She told me that she had started seeing a counsellor for weekly sessions and it was going well. The counsellor (a woman) had told her that it was time to stop wallowing in misery and to try and change her life. This sounded rather different from my style so I asked whether they talked about any of the things which Louise and I had talked about.

'Oh yes,' she said. 'We talk about my childhood and my father and, of course, my mother. And we talk about you!' She promised that she would now fill in my questionnaire, but so far I have not received it.

JENNIFER. Jennifer did send the questionnaire back, very promptly, and this is what she wrote:

165

'In the main my life is tremendously better than it was during all the years when my nerves were being treated. This is partly because of various changes in my life and partly because I have come to terms with various aspects of my life. I would say that the outcome was helpful. The experience of it was hampered to some small degree by the fact that the therapist was not a stranger. I had already been a patient for a number of years, I imagined you had some concept, if not knowledge, of my family. In the context that I would continue to be a patient, these sort of things inhibit one's 'opening up' – the continuity works against this. I do not believe that it has altered the direction of my life, but then how can one ever know? I recall at the time being impressed by the generosity of the offer of therapy which, in itself, must have contributed to healing. I recall thinking that if I went much further down that road I might find myself having to look for another GP and weighing up the two opposite outcomes. I would say that your role was changing and I suppose I wanted to retain the role I would need the longest. I doubt this was totally conscious at the time.'

This was a very thoughtful response and it made me think too. Jennifer was the only patient to say that the fact that I was also the family doctor was inhibiting. She also suggested that she might have opened up more and perhaps made more progress with a stranger. I did offer to refer her back to her psychotherapist at one stage, but she did not seem to want that. ('I feel ashamed about needing her again.') I feel slightly chastened and put in my place at being valued more as a GP than as a psychotherapist: but it is nice to be valued for something.

How has Jennifer fared according to the six criteria? She is obviously enjoying her job which seems to be very stimulating and up to her intellectual expectations. I do not know much about her social life; only that she is resigned to doing without a life partner. She never really risked becoming dependent on me, but she did have a tendency to reach for the bottle when she felt lonely. I have not dared ask whether this still happens. I did not seek her out for a face to face interview, feeling that her replies to the questionnaire suggested that she would not want that. Nevertheless I find the tone of what she has written with its sense of peace and balance quite reassuring.

EPILOGUE

That concludes the follow-up and evaluation. I have used the six criteria as a background to be borne in mind rather than attempting to score each patient on each criterion in turn. No marks have been awarded, there are no winners and no losers, and I certainly do not want to award myself any points. I view the patients rather as if they were my children, now grown up. I am acutely interested in their progress and their affairs; I take a fierce pride and pleasure in their achievements and I share in their disappointments. Regretfully I have to note the ambitions that were unachieved, and now look as though they never will be achieved. Like a parent I may have to come to terms with the fact that some of them were my ambitions anyway, and not theirs. Like a parent, I always enjoy hearing news of my 'children', and when possible being in their company. I miss the ones who are far away and never write.

I still see one psychotherapy patient weekly as well as my six-weekly sessions with Margaret. Meanwhile General Practice in Britain is undergoing a major upheaval and seems likely to become epidemiological or population-centred in emphasis, rather than focusing on the individual and his or her uniqueness. Like many of my colleagues I regret these changes, and feel that they have been imposed on us by a government that has little understanding of our patients' real needs. I can only hope that with all the health checks to perform and the statistics to collect, I will still feel able, at the end of the day, to settle down and give my full attention to the patient with the Last Appointment.

BIBLIOGRAPHY

Alexander, F. and French, J.M. (1946). *Psychoanalytic Therapy: Principles and Application.* Ronald Press, New York.

Balint, M. (1957). *The Doctor, his Patient and the Illness.* Pitman, London.

Balint, M. (1968). *The Basic Fault.* Tavistock/Routledge, London.

Balint, M. and Balint, E. (1961). *Psychotherapeutic Techniques in Medicine.* Tavistock, London.

Balint, M. and Norell, J.S., (eds) (1973) *Six Minutes for the Patient.* Tavistock, London.

Crown, S. and Crisp, A.H. (1966) *A short clinical self rating scale for psychoneurotic patients.* Brit. J. Psychiat. 112. 917-23.

Dinnage, R. (1988). *One to One: Experiences of Psychotherapy.* Viking Penguin, London.

Earll, L. and Kincy, J. (1982) *Clinical psychology in General Practice: a Controlled Trial Evaluation.* J. Roy. Coll. Gen. Pract. 31, 32-37.

Ferenczi, S. (1932) *Clinical Diaries.* Translated by Michael Balint and Nicola Jackson, edited by Judith Dupont (1988). Harvard University Press, Cambridge, Mass., USA, and London.

Frank, J. (1974) *Persuasion and Healing. A comparative study of psychotherapy.* Schocken Books, New York.

Freud, S. (1912). *'Recommendations to Physicians Practising Psychoanalysis.'* Standard Edition of the Complete Psychological Works of Sigmund Freud, 12. Hogarth Press, London.

Freud, S. (1917). *Introductory Lectures on Psychoanalysis.* Standard Edition, 16.

Freud, S. (1937). *'Analysis Terminable and Interminable.'* Standard Edition, 23.

Goldberg, D. and Huxley, P. (1980). *Mental Illness in the Community.* Tavistock, London.

Heiman, P. (1950). *'On Countertransference,'* International Journal of Psychoanalysis, 31, 81-4.

Ives, G. (1979). *Psychological treatment in General Practice.* Journal of the Royal College of General Practitioners. 29. 343-351.

Jones, E. (1953-7). *The Life and Work of Sigmund Freud.* Hogarth Press, London.

Klein, M. (1946). *'Notes on some Schizoid Mechanisms,'* In Envy and Gratitude and other works 1944-63. (1975). Hogarth Press, London.

Lomas, P. (1987). *The Limits of Interpretation: What's wrong with Psychoanalysis?* Penguin Books, London.

McLeod, J. (1988). *The Work of Counsellors in General Practice.* Occasional Paper No 37, Royal College of General Practitioners, London.

Malcolm, J. (1988). *Psychoanalysis: the Impossible Profession.* Picador, London.

Mellinger, G., Balter, M., Manheimer, D., Cisin, I. and Parry, H. (1978). *'Psychic Distress, Life Crisis, and Use of Psychotherapeutic Medications,'* Archives of General Psychiatry, 35, 1045-52.

Obholzer, K. (1980). *The Wolf Man Sixty Years Later.* Routledge and Kegan Paul, London.

Roazen, P. (1971). *Freud and his Followers.* Allen Lane, London.

Rogers, C. (1961). *On Becoming a Person.* Constable, London.

Samuel, O. (1989). *'How Doctors Learn in Balint Groups'.* Family Practice, 6, 108-113.

Skegg, D.C.G., Doll, R. and Perry, J. (1975). *'Use of Medicines in General Practice',* British Medical Journal, 1, 1561-3.

Storr, A. (1960). *The Integrity of the Personality.* Penguin Books, London.

Storr, A. (1989). *Freud.* Oxford University Press, Oxford.

Suttie, I. (1935). *The Origins of Love and Hate.* Routledge and Kegan Paul, London.

Winnicott, D.W. (1962). *'The Aims of Psycho-analytical Treatment',* in The Maturational Process and the Facilitating Environment (1987), Hogarth Press, London.

Winnicott, D.W. (1963). *'Psychiatric Disorders in terms of Infantile Maturational Processes,'* in The Maturational Process and the Facilitating Environment (1987), Hogarth Press, London.

ACKNOWLEDGEMENTS

The author gratefully acknowledges permission to use quotations from the following sources:

Dinnage, Rosemary. *One to One: Experiences of Psychotherapy* (1988) by permission of Penguin Books Ltd.
Freud, Sigmund. The Standard Edition of the Complete Psychological Works of Sigmund Freud, translated and edited by James Strachey (1955) by permission of Chatto and Windus, The Institute of Psychoanalysis and The Hogarth Press.
Ferenczi, Sandor. The Clinical Diaries of Sandor Ferenczi, translated by Michael Balint and Nicola Jackson, edited by Judith Dupont (1988) by permission of Harvard University Press.
Lomas, Peter. *The Limits of Interpretation: What's Wrong with Psychoanalysis?* (1987) by permission of Penguin Books Ltd.
Malcolm, Janet. *Psychoanalysis: the Impossible Profession* (1988) by permission of Pan Books Ltd.
Roazen, Paul. *Freud and his Followers* (1971) by permission of Allen Lane, Penguin Books Ltd.
Rogers, Carl. *On Becoming a Person* (1971) by permission of Constable and Co Ltd.
Storr, Anthony. *The Integrity of the Personality* (1960) by permission of Penguin Books Ltd.

171

Storr, Anthony. *Freud* (1989) by permission of Oxford University Press.
Winnicott, D.W. *The Maturational Process and the Facilitating Environment* (1987) by permission of Chatto and Windus.